Informed Consent

A Tutorial

Informed Consent

A Tutorial

T. M. Grundner, Ed. D.

NHP NATIONAL HEALTH PUBLISHING

Copyright © 1986 by
Rynd Communications
99 Painters Mill Road
Owings Mills, MD 21117

All rights reserved. No
parts of this publication
may be reproduced in any
form except by prior
written permission from
the publisher.

Printed in the United States of America
First Printing
ISBN: 0-932500-57-9
LC: 86-62615

KF
3827
.I5
G78
1986

To William F. O'Neill, Ph.D. and
John A. Carpenter, Ph.D.

"To consider dear to me as my parents him who taught me this art..."

Hippocratic Oath

Contents

About the Author *ix*
Introduction *xi*
To the Reader *xvii*

Chapter 1   A Brief Historical Overview *1*

Chapter 2   The Consent Process *11*

Chapter 3   Consent Form Content: The Beginning Section *39*

Chapter 4   Consent Form Content: The Middle Section *59*

Chapter 5   Consent Form Content: The Ending *91*

Chapter 6   Consent Form Content: Additional Elements *123*

Chapter 7   Altering or Waiving Consent *143*

Chapter 8   Working with Special Populations *163*

Chapter 9   A Final Summing-Up *175*

Appendix A   45 CFR 46: The Federal Regulations Governing Human Experimentation *189*

Appendix B   A Protocol for Determining Consent Form Readability *219*

Appendix C   Sample Consent Form *225*

Appendix D   A Consent Checklist *227*

About the Author

T.M. Grundner is an assistant professor and Director of the Division of Medical Education and Informatics in the Department of Family Medicine at Case Western Reserve University School of Medicine in Cleveland, Ohio. A native of Detroit, he received his undergraduate degree in psychology from Eastern Michigan University, a master's degree in human learning from the Institute for Behavioral Research in Silver Springs, Maryland, a second master's in education from the University of Southern California, and a doctorate in educational philosophy, also from USC. He has taught widely in the area of research ethics with particular reference to the informed consent process, and his articles have appeared in journals ranging from the *American Psychologist* to the *New England Journal of Medicine*. In addition to his work in this area, Dr. Grundner is a widely recognized authority in the use of computerized communications systems for delivering community health education.

Introduction

The history of human experimentation is a fascinating one. It is filled with brilliant discoveries, bitter rivalries, and drama that is made all the more penetrating by the fact that it did not flow from a fiction writer's pen.

The history of the ethical issues that surround human experimentation is no less fascinating. As you will see in Chapter 1, it is filled with genuine heroes, unbelievable villains, and thousands of persons who were somewhere in between. It has a certain poignancy to it that is quite different from what you might find in a straightforward history of science. It is different, I believe, because of the direct personal relevance it has for all of us.

Let me put it another way. Only a handful of people are remembered on the pages of scientific history. Yet no one, be they Nobel Prize winners or first-year students, can avoid the ethical issues inherent in their work. When you started college, you had a choice as to what profession you wished to enter. You chose one of the sciences. Later on, you chose (or will choose) a specialty and, within that specialty, you chose (or will choose) a particular area of interest. Along the way, you had choices and you made them.

With regard to the area of professional ethics, however, you have no choice. Whether you wish to become an ethicist in your particular discipline is not at issue. You are one. You became one the minute you joined a profession. The only thing that's at issue now is whether you are going to be a good ethicist or a bad one.

It is virtually impossible to pursue any of the sciences in a value-free context. This is especially true when human research is involved. You cannot use a human being in an experimental setting--even in the most innocuous of experiments--without, at some point, asking yourself, "Ought I to be doing this, in this way, to this person, at this time?" The moment the word "ought" is muttered, you have entered the realm of ethics.

It is toward the goal of creating more good "ethicists" that this book is dedicated.

The Rules of the Game

There are numerous complex and controversial ethical issues surrounding the field of human experimentation--issues that have tied professional philosophers in knots for years. We, however, will not be soaring to such lofty heights in this volume. For us the task is much easier. At this introductory level, for all practical intents and purposes, what constitutes "ethical conduct" is defined for us by statute. More specifically, it is defined for us in the *Code of Federal Regulations*, Title 45, Part 46, Section 46.101 to 46.409 or, as it is more affectionately known--45 CFR 46. We will be basing this volume on the last revision of it on March 8, 1983.

These regulations, although not without controversy themselves, contain the last word with regard to what can and cannot be done with human subjects. They apply to all research work funded by Department of Health and Human Services (HHS) monies conducted on human beings in any discipline and, in general, provide the standard by which the ethics of all research work is judged, no matter what its funding source. For our purposes, it will be the Bible, and for this reason I have had it reprinted in Appendix A.

Among the many controversial sections within 45 CFR 46 is one which some people think allows for the automatic exemption of most projects in the educational, social, and behavioral sciences. I want to clear up this misconception before we go any further because nothing could be further from reality.

In the most recent revision of 45 CFR 46, changes were made which created certain categories of "exempted research." In other words, the federal government declared that, as far as it was concerned, certain types of research work would be considered exempt from the regulations. These categories included certain types of educational research and certain types of survey, interview, and observational research--all mainstays of the biomedical as well as the social and behavioral sciences. The government didn't say, however, that these categories *had* to be exempt, nor did it specify what procedures needed to be followed to determine if any given project was to fall into one or more of these exempted categories. It is here that the confusion and misunderstandings arise.

Every institution conducting human research work of any volume has a group of people known generically as an Institutional Review Board (IRB). This IRB reviews all research conducted at that institution for its conformity to the federal regulations. It is, in effect, the interpreter and enforcer of 45 CFR 46 at the local level.

In some areas, the federal guidelines give the IRBs virtually no choice as to how things will be done. In other areas, they do. These guidelines do give each IRB some latitude in deciding what internal procedures the group will follow to gather the information necessary to make its determinations. The "exempted categories" might be exempt as far as the federal government is concerned, but there is nothing to say that the local IRBs can't require researchers to fill out all the forms and provide all the documentation required of any other project to determine if their particular project indeed qualifies for exemption. In overwhelming numbers, this is exactly what the IRBs have done.

One study, conducted approximately one year after the revised federal regulations were released,[1] indicated that 80%-90% of the IRBs (depending on the specific category) chose *not* to automatically exempt the "exempted categories" and chose to keep them under at least some kind of review. The projects were federally exempt, but you couldn't tell the difference as far as the IRB procedures were concerned.

It is possible that you are, or will be, at an institution that has granted automatic exemption from any IRB review to these types of projects. It is possible, but given the data presented above, not likely. This volume will therefore assume that all research--including research in the exempted categories--must be able to withstand a full IRB review.

In addition, in almost all cases, this volume will take a strict constructionist approach to the rest of the regulations. It will take the position (considered radical in some quarters) that the regulations actually mean what they so clearly say.

Finally, as you've probably guessed from the title, we will be focusing on only those portions of 45 CFR 46 dealing with how to design, evaluate, and administer an "informed consent." There are other federal regulations for drug research that also deal with informed consent, but we will not touch on them here. While they may closely parallel those regulations I will discuss, they are not exactly the same. If you are involved in drug research, you should follow the most recent Food and Drug Administration guidelines.

Virtually everything in this book will be based on 45 CFR 46. Given the nature of these regulations, however, a certain element of personal interpretation is inevitable. I'll try to distinguish between my interpretation and strict regulatory intent by referencing all elements that are drawn directly from the regulations.*

A Word About IRBs

A few paragraphs ago, I mentioned that the term IRB stood for the words "Institutional Review Board" and that this was a committee of people who were empowered to review all research conducted at a given institution for its conformity to 45 CFR 46. If your institution receives money from any branch of the Department of Health and Human Services for research with human

---

* Throughout the book, the numbers you see in brackets refer to sections within 45 CFR 46, reprinted in Appendix A. Thus, if you were to see [46.116(a)(1)], it would be referring you to section 46.116, paragraph (a), subparagraph (1).

subjects, then you either have such a committee set up, or your institution has an agreement with another institution to use their committee.

Now before you go rushing to your phone book, keep in mind that the name Institutional Review Board is a generic one intended to cover all such committees. Your particular board might go under a different name, such as the Human Subjects Committee or Committee on Research Ethics, but if you ask around you'll find it.

These committees are not only empowered to enforce 45 CFR 46 and interpret it for *you*, but they are *themselves* very much controlled by it. The regulations stipulate very precisely the composition of the IRB [46.107], its functions [46.108], the records it must keep [46.115], and a whole host of other matters that influence its work [46.103(b)(4)]. Included in these requirements is one that says the IRB must file what is called an "assurance" with HHS which stipulates exactly how the board will operate. No projects can be funded unless this assurance is in place and unless the project has met with IRB approval [46.103(b)].

Strictly speaking, 45 CFR 46 pertains only to research funded, in whole or in part, by HHS monies. Many researchers have bridled over the fact that they have had to submit their research for review when it was funded by someone else--a private foundation, for example. The reason for requiring these submissions is that tucked away in the assurance requirements is a clause that requires the IRB to specify what principles it will use to govern non-HHS funded research at its institution [46.103(b)(1)]. Most IRBs took the path of least resistance when they filed their assurance, and said "45 CFR 46." That's why virtually all research, including theses and dissertations, must come under IRB review at most institutions.

How extensive are the powers of the IRB? In point of fact, they are nearly total. It is the IRB that must certify your research to HHS; that is, officially notify the Department that your project has been reviewed according to the regulations and according to the terms of the assurance, and that everything is okay [46.102(h)]. Very simply, it works like this: no certification, no money [46.103(b)]. Furthermore, should you decide not to comply with its determinations, the IRB is required by law (remember, 45 CFR 46 is a federal law) to report you to the appropriate institutional officials and/or to HHS. HHS can and will immediately stop your funding until the matter is cleared up or it may terminate your project completely [46.113]. Needless to say, such an eventuality is rarely viewed as career enhancing. Finally, if the IRB says no to a project, there is no one in your institution who can overrule it, so don't even ask [46.112].

I realize that this paints a pretty bleak picture of your friendly IRB. It's not meant to. Indeed, some of the most helpful people you will ever encounter serve on these committees. In most cases, they will go far out of their way to guide you through the review process, and truly, you should rely on them for this purpose. Their job is not to harass you; it is to help, and they will. But you have to keep in mind that they, too, have constraints. They *must* do what the regulations say. HHS isn't kidding about this stuff.

What, then, must the IRB do? It must see that the provisions of 45 CFR 46 are honored which, in many ways, is what this entire book is about--especially as it pertains to informed consent. In addition to the consent issue, the IRB will generally review your research with regard to a number of other criteria as well. Briefly stated, these criteria are as follows [46.111]:

1. That the risks to the subjects are minimized.
2. That the risks to the subjects are reasonable in relation to anticipated benefits.
3. That the selection of subjects is equitable.
4. That an informed consent will be sought from each prospective subject or the subject's legally authorized representative.
5. That the informed consent will be properly documented.
6. That, where appropriate, adequate provisions are made for the safety of the subjects.
7. That, where appropriate, adequate provisions are made for the privacy of the subject and the confidentiality of the data.

When you think about it, those are not unreasonable demands.

Some Definitions

Before we go into any more specifics, there are some definitions we need to get out of the way. They are important because they will help you to determine whether the project you are thinking about undertaking is indeed considered "research" for the purposes of these regulations.

Research will refer to any systematic investigation designed to develop or contribute to generalizable knowledge. This, by the way, also includes activities that may not normally go under the title of research *per se*. For example, some "demonstration" and "service" programs may well include "research" activities under this definition [46.102(e)].

A *human subject* is any living individual about whom an investigator (whether professional or student) conducting research obtains (1) data through *intervention* or *interaction* with the individual, or (2) identifiable *private information* [46.102(f)].

Okay, now what might those italicized words mean?

An *intervention* includes both physical procedures by which data are gathered and manipulations of the subject or his environment that might be performed for research purposes. An *interaction* includes any communication or interpersonal contact between an investigator and a subject. *Private information* includes information about behavior that occurs in a context in which the individual can reasonably expect that no observation or recording is taking place, and information which has been provided for specific purposes other than research and which the individual can reasonably expect will not be made public. To fall under these guidelines, this private information must be individually identifiable. In other words, if the investigator could readily identify who the subject is or if the subject could be associated with the data in some way, it would fall into this category [46.102(f)].

Finally, this is a definition we will come across many times in this volume, namely *minimal risk*. Minimal risk means that the risks of harm anticipated in the proposed study are not greater, considering probability and magnitude, than those ordinarily encountered in daily life or during the performance of routine physical or psychological examinations or tests [46.102(g)].

If your project does not constitute "research" or involve "human subjects" as either term is defined here, then you need go no further. These particular regulations do not apply to you.

Keep in mind that many federal agencies besides HHS have something to say about research with human subjects, as do many state and local governments. To find out whether any of them has something to say about your particular project, contact your local IRB. We in no way want to leave you with the impression that this book represents the final, definitive, and ultimate word on what you can and cannot do in an informed consent.

The final word is contained in the regulations as they are interpreted by your local IRB. Do not hesitate to read the regulations for yourself and to utilize your IRB if you have any questions at all. It will be happy to explain how any portion of these regulations are being applied at your particular location.

So, that's about it. You and this book have now been properly introduced.

Oh yes, one last word of caution. This text is written in a way that might be unfamiliar to many of you and may require a bit of explanation. Be sure to read the section entitled "To the Reader" for details.

Reference

1. Grundner, T. M. "DHHS Human Subjects Protection: The New Regulations Revisited." *Health Matrix* 1, no. 2 (1983):37-41.

To the Reader

You may find that this book is written differently from other texts you have read. With the exception of the first and last chapters, each chapter begins with a narrative text that constitutes the "chapter opening." This is followed by the first in a series of "situations." Following each situation will be a question.

Your job is to read the chapter opening, then read the first situation and choose an answer to the question that follows it. The answer you choose will refer you to another page which will tell you whether you are right or wrong and why. This page, in turn, will refer you to another page and so on through the book. By following these instructions, the material will adjust itself to your needs and you can proceed without being distracted by unnecessary explanations.

Nothing to it. Let's begin.

Turn to page 1.

Chapter 1
A Brief Historical Overview

I swear by Apollo the Physician, by Aesculapius, Hygeia, and Panacea, and I take to witness all the gods, all the goddesses, to keep according to my ability and my judgment the following Oath:

To consider dear to me as my parents him who taught me this art; to live in common with him and if necessary to share my goods with him; to look upon his children as my own brothers, to teach them this art if they so desire without fee or written promise; to impart to my sons and the sons of the master who taught me and the disciples who have enrolled themselves and have agreed to the rules of the profession, but to these alone, the precepts and the instruction. I will prescribe regimen for the good of my patients according to my ability and my judgment and never do harm to anyone. To please no one will I prescribe a deadly drug, nor give advice which may cause his death. Nor will I give a woman a pessary to procure abortion. But I will preserve the purity of my life and my art. I will not cut for stone, even for patients in whom the disease is manifest; I will leave this operation to be performed by practitioners (specialists in this art). In every house where I come I will enter only for the good of my patients, keeping myself far from all intentional ill-doing and all seduction, and especially from the pleasures of love with women or with men, be they free or slaves. All that may come to my knowledge in the exercise of my profession or outside of my profession or in daily commerce with men, which ought not to be spread abroad, I will keep secret and will never reveal. If I keep this oath faithfully, may I enjoy my life and practice my art, respected by all men and in all times; but if I swerve from it or violate it, may the reverse be my lot.[1]

Early Movements: Rhetoric vs. Reality

The above statement is, of course, the Hippocratic Oath. While the writing is probably not actually that of the 5th Century B.C. physician, Hippocrates, it clearly expresses the values for which he and his guild were known. These values formed the core of early medical and ethical thinking and can still be seen today in many of the belief structures of the biomedical and social sciences.

The oath remained intact for generations, being passed on from father to son, master to student. It was not long, however, before chinks began to appear in medicine's idealistic armor--especially when it came to human experimentation. Compare, for example, the idealism of the Hippocratic Oath with the reality of ancient and medieval "experimental protocol." Claude Bernard, in 1856, writes:

> We are told that the Kings of Persia delivered men condemned to death to their physicians, so that they might perform on them vivisections useful to science. According to Galen, Attalus III (Philometer), who reigned at Pergamum, one hundred thirty seven years before Jesus Christ, experimented with poisons and antidotes on criminals condemned to death. Celsus recalls and approves the vivisection which Herophilus and Erasistratus performed on criminals with the Ptolemies' consent. It is not cruel, he says, to inflict on a few criminals, sufferings which may benefit multitudes of innocent people throughout all centuries. The Grand Duke of Tuscany had a criminal given over to the professor of anatomy, Fallopius, at Pisa, with permission to kill or dissect him at pleasure. As the criminal had a quartan fever, Fallopius wished to investigate the effects of opium on the paroxysms. He administered two drams of opium during an intermission; death occurred after the second experiment. Similar instances have occasionally recurred, and the story is well known of the archer of Meudon who was pardoned because a nephrotomy (i.e., a surgical incision into the kidney) was successfully performed on him.[2]

Throughout the Middle Ages the shape of what constitutes the customary and proper practices of a physician was beginning to emerge. No significant references were being made to human experimentation, however. Until about the 19th century, medicine was considered more of an art form than a science. Because so little was occurring in the way of scientific inquiry, little notice was taken of the ethical issues that might surround the use of human subjects. Once these ethical issues were raised, however, the pace of ethical development quickened.

In 1803 Thomas Percival, writing in what may have been the world's first textbook on medical ethics, pointed out that, in general, research is supposed to be conducted for the public good--especially the good of the poor.[3] Yet, he argued, even though such experimental work is frequently done under extreme circumstances, researchers are still obliged to maintain the highest standards of practice.

William Beaumont, the renowned American physician and researcher, in 1883 drew up his own personal code of research ethics in which he argued for the importance of methodological soundness in human research studies, the voluntary consent of the subject, and the right of the subject to withdraw and terminate his role in the experiment at any time.[4]

Claude Bernard, regarded by many as the father of modern experimental medicine, took Beaumont one step further, at least in terms of eloquence and succinctness. In 1856 he wrote:

Christian morals forbid only one thing, doing harm to one's neighbors. So, among experiments that may be tried on man, those that can only do harm are forbidden, those that are harmless are permissible, and those that may do good are obligatory.[5]

Once again, however, despite these lofty sentiments, a closer examination of the experimental practices of the day reveals a considerable gap between rhetoric and reality.

The Russian physician, Vikentii Smidovich, who wrote under the pseudonym of V.V. Veressayev, devoted a full chapter of his memoirs to a blistering attack on the ethics of his colleagues, especially those who conducted syphilis experiments in the 1850s. After presenting a case by case litany of abuses, including the intentional infection of young women to study the course of the disease, he wrote:

One would suppose that the mere fact of publication of such experiments would make their repetition utterly impossible, the first to attempt anything of the kind being cast out forever from the medical corporation. But, unfortunately, this is not so. With heads proudly erect, these bizarre disciples of science proceed upon their way without encountering any effective opposition, either from their colleagues or from the medical press . . . [6]

But sentiments similar to Veressayev's, while presumably felt in other quarters, rarely took the form of published attack. One major reason for this was the lack of standardized guidelines to which the behavior of a researcher could be compared. This deficiency remained until 1948 and, even then, changed only as a result of one of the greatest horror stories of all time. The vehicle for uncovering this horror was a courtroom in Nuremberg, Germany.

The Modern Era: Tragedy and Progress

If the early development of ethical thinking with regard to human research can be characterized as one of laudable rhetoric and unconscionable practice, the modern one can be characterized as one of progress fueled by tragedy. The first of these tragedies was laid bare by the Nuremberg Tribunal following World War II.

The Nazi medical cases, generically known as *United States v. Brandt*,[7] focused the world's attention on the kinds of horrors that can occur when research ethics go unspecified and uncontrolled. Detailed in these proceedings were experiments on high altitude endurance, where subjects were placed unprotected in low pressure chambers that could duplicate the pressures and temperatures of high altitude flight; freezing experiments, where subjects were forced to remain in tanks of ice water for periods of up to three hours to find the best method of treating people who had been severely chilled or frozen; disease experiments, where subjects were deliberately injected with malaria, epidemic jaundice, spotted fever, and other diseases in order to test vaccines; antibiotics experiments, where subjects were wounded and then intentionally infected with various bacteria to test the effectiveness of the then new drug sulfanilamide; and finally, poison experiments where subjects were given various poisons merely to see how long it would take for them to die.

In the end, 15 defendants had been convicted of criminal responsibility in the deaths of hundreds of "subjects," seven had been acquitted, and a series of basic principles had been laid down " . . . to satisfy moral, ethical and legal concepts."[8]

The Tribunal eventually issued these basic principles in a document which stated, among other things, that in all research work with human subjects the voluntary consent of the participant was essential; that the study should yield fruitful results for the good of society; that it should be based on prior animal research; that it should avoid all unnecessary suffering, injury, or death; that the degree of risk should never outweigh the importance of the study; that the study should be undertaken only by qualified persons; and that either the scientist or the subject can and should bring the study to a halt if continuation of the experiment is untenable or dangerous.[9]

These principles soon became known as the "Nuremberg Code" and provided the world with a set of specific ethical standards to which the research community could be held accountable. The way was finally clear for the systematic ethical analysis of research; researchers, in turn, finally had a definite statement of ethical norms to which they could tailor their activities. Virtually every major ethical code or set of human research guidelines that have been developed since then have been based, in whole or in part, on these principles.

From today's perspective one might assume that these Nuremberg principles caused an immediate sensation in the scientific community. They did not. Indeed, they were virtually ignored in most quarters until the 1960s.

This is not to say, however, that work on ethical standardization did not continue, for it did. The problem was that, at the time, there was no pressure on either the scientific or political communities for these principles to become anything more than abstract sentiments. The Nuremberg Code, for example, had absolutely no authority behind it. It was merely a set of recommendations buried in millions of war documents.

The first step in the process of giving teeth to the Nuremberg principles came in 1953 when the U.S. Public Health Service (PHS) issued a document called "Group Consideration of Clinical Research Procedures Deviating from Accepted Medical Practice or Involving Unusual Hazard."[10] For the first time, a governmental agency had gone on record as being concerned with the issue of research ethics and had demonstrated this concern by writing a policy statement about it. The policy was not a particularly strong one, but it was an official policy, and it was a precedent.

The PHS policy essentially dealt with three major areas. First, it proposed that researchers show more concern over what constitutes acceptable and unacceptable subject risk when designing an experiment. Second, it raised the issue of how much subjects should be told when they give their consent to participate in a project. Finally, and most importantly, it raised for the first time the idea that research should be subject to some sort of ethical review. This latter idea proved to be seminal to the development of the peer review (IRB) system we have today.

Despite the importance of these concepts, the overall policy was weak because it failed to take two very important steps. First, while it recommended peer review, such review was not required. The ethical monitoring of a research project remained in the hands of the individual researcher. Second, the policy pertained *only* to intramural programs, that is, programs that were being conducted by PHS employees.

The year 1962 brought the issue of research ethics to the foreground once more and, as with the Nuremberg Code, it took a tragedy to stimulate the next major advance in ethical regulation. In 1957, a West German pharmaceutical firm, Chemie Grunenthal, began marketing a new tranquilizer. It was billed as safe, nontoxic, free of side effects, and particularly good for use with pregnant women. Its trade name was Contergan, and mothers in 46 countries around the world happily took the drug. Before the drug--whose generic name was thalidomide--could be removed from the market, over 8,000 horribly deformed babies had been born.

The United States was largely spared this disaster. Because of the skepticism and stubbornness of one official in the FDA, the drug was never approved for distribution. It was a close call, however, and Congress decided to take a closer look at safeguards being used in the testing and approval of pharmaceuticals. They also decided to look at the safeguards that were in place to protect the subjects of those tests. The result was the 1962 Drug Amendments Act, sometimes known as the Kefauver-Harris Bill,[11] and once again the subject of ethical protocol was addressed. The major ethical feature of the Act was the demand that the informed consent of all drug study subjects be obtained. This was something that at the time was not a routine procedure. Unfortunately, the policy also left three loopholes. First, it was not necessary to obtain the consent of the subject where the *investigator* felt it was not feasible. Second, the only research covered by the policy was research on new drugs. Third, there were no specifications as to how that consent was to be obtained. In short, it was a good idea, but like other policies, it really had no widespread authority.

As it took the Nazi horrors to generate the Nuremberg Code and the thalidomide tragedy to spawn the Kefauver-Harris bill, it took yet another instance of research abuse to promote the next major development. In July of 1963, three doctors at the Jewish Chronic Disease Hospital in New York injected live cancer cells into 22 elderly subjects without informing them. The result was a major legal battle and a public furor that raged for months. This incident gave the Public Health Service the impetus necessary to again revise its policy on the protection of human subjects.

Basically, PHS took some of the best features of the Nuremberg Code, its own 1954 policy, the Kefauver-Harris Bill, added a few new touches and combined them into a coherent whole. The final standards were released in 1966.[12] Included among its provisions were (1) that committees should be established to review proposed research; (2) that the rights and welfare of the subjects must always be protected; (3) that the consent process must be monitored; (4) that the risks of the research must not outweigh its benefits; (5) that the research should undergo continued monitoring; and (6) that documentation must be kept on all of the above. In addition, and perhaps most importantly, it was specified that this policy was to apply to *all* institutions receiving monies from PHS.

The historical importance of this document can be seen because shortly thereafter, it made the basis for an even more extensive policy issued by the Department of Health, Education and Welfare (HEW).[13] HEW not only ratified the PHS provisions but set up specific mechanisms to force compliance. Institutions that were not in compliance stood the risk of losing all HEW and PHS funding.

Following close on the heels of HEW was the Food and Drug Administration with a similar policy.[14] In effect, within a few short years, virtually every research organization in the country was brought under extensive *mandatory* ethical guidelines--guidelines that frame the basis for the way research is conducted today. For this reason, these regulations require a much closer review.

From HEW to HHS: Consolidation and Controversy

On December 1, 1971, the Department of Health, Education and Welfare issued an innocuous-looking yellow booklet entitled "The Institutional Guide to DHEW Policy on the Protection of Human Rights."[15] It was perhaps the most significant piece of regulatory work ever done in the area of human research. Probably its most important contribution, however, was to functionally implement the peer review process, a concept that had been discussed since the 1954 PHS guidelines but had never been acted upon. Essentially, it required every institution receiving HEW monies for human research (which was just about everyone) to create a central committee to monitor the ethical integrity of its research projects.

These committees, generically known as Institutional Review Boards (IRBs), were to examine all projects being submitted by members of that institution for funding and were to provide assurance to HEW that they were being conducted in an ethically permissible manner. What constituted the "ethically permissible" was detailed in the policy and emphasized the calculation of risk-benefit ratios (i.e., that the benefits of the research should outweigh the risks to the subjects) and the careful collection of documented informed consents.

The system was a work of bureaucratic genius. As discussed earlier, one of the major problems with ethical policy in the past had been the issue of enforcement. It was a touchy matter. Even if a tight policy were to be created, what would happen to those who broke it? Or, an even tougher question: how would you know if it had been broken in the first place? Would the government have an army of investigators lurking around thousands of laboratories? Would there be an "Ethical FBI" to follow up on rumors of conspiratorial violation? No, indeed. With this policy HEW simply provided the institutions with the guidelines and said, in effect, "You enforce it and, if violations occur, both the researcher *and the institution* could have their eligibility removed for all future HEW research monies involving human subjects." That last clause clearly got the attention of university and hospital administrators. Whether the individual researcher liked it or not, ethical adherence had suddenly become a very serious matter.

That the policy was taken seriously, however, is not the same thing as saying that everyone agreed with it. There was a great deal of pressure to step back and give this whole area considerably more thought. Accordingly, on July 12th, 1974 Congress passed Public Law 93-348 which established a blue ribbon panel of experts to

> (i) conduct a comprehensive investigation and study to identify the basic ethical principles which should underlie the conduct of biomedical and behavioral research involving human subjects,

(ii) develop guidelines which should be followed in such research to assure that it is conducted in accordance with such principles, and

(iii) make recommendations to The Secretary (of DHEW) for such administrative action as may be appropriate to apply such guidelines to biomedical and behavioral research conducted or supported under programs administered by The Secretary.[16]

The result of this legislation was the creation of the National Commission for the Protection of Human Subjects of Biomedical and Behavioral Research--one of the finest examples of a functional governmental commission on record.

By the time the Commission had finished its work in October of 1978, it had produced 10 sets of recommendations ranging in scope from a set of general philosophical principles to guide researchers, to detailed policy recommendations on how to ethically conduct research work with groups as diverse as children, prisoners, and the mentally infirm. In addition, for each set of recommendations it produced appendices which are still among the finest single sources of information on research ethics and its collateral issues.

The Secretary of HEW (now called the Secretary of Health and Human Services) took the Commission recommendations and converted them into a "notice of proposed rulemaking" and published them for public comment in the August 14, 1979 edition of the *Federal Register*.[17]

Eventually, over 500 comments were received. The final regulations were altered according to this response and according to the decisions of the HHS staff members working on the project. They were issued in final form on January 26, 1981 as 45 CFR 46.[18]

In the last few years, the HHS regulations have become the "industry standard." While technically they apply only to federally funded research, at last count, over 96% of IRBs were applying them to all research projects whether they were funded by federal money or not.[19] To put it another way, it is almost impossible for a person to conduct research using human subjects in any one of the sciences without, at some point or another, coming into contact with an IRB that is wielding the federal regulations. Indeed, that is one reason this book was written.

Another problem still remains to be solved. It is one thing to say that the federal standards obtain for almost all institutionally conducted research, and quite another to insure that all researchers are well aware of what those regulations require of them.

In a 1983 study of behavioral science IRBs, it was found that over 27% of the applications received were initially rejected. The most common reason given for rejection (92.7%) was because the consent form or the consent procedure was flawed.[20]

With *that* kind of data in mind, we begin our study of informed consent.

References

1. *Stedman's Medical Dictionary*, 24th ed., s.v. "Hippocratic Oath."
2. Reiser, S.J., A.J. Dyck, and W.J. Curran. *Ethics in Medicine: Historical Perspectives and Contemporary Concerns*. Cambridge, MA: MIT Press, 1977.
3. Beecher, H.K. *Research and the Individual*. Boston: Little, Brown and Co., 1970.
4. *Ibid.*
5. *Ibid.*
6. Veressayev, V.V. *The Memoirs of a Physician*. Translated by Simeon Linden. New York: Knopf, 1916.
7. United States Adjutant General's Department. *Final Report to the Secretary of the Army on the Nuremberg War Crimes Trials under Control Council Law No. 10*. Washington, DC: U.S. Government Printing Office, 1948.
8. *Ibid.*
9. *Ibid.*
10. Gray, B.H. *Human Subjects in Medical Experimentation*. New York: John Wiley & Sons, 1975.
11. P.L. 87-781, 21 U.S.C. 355.
12. Gray. *Human Subjects in Medical Experimentation*.
13. *Institutional Guide to DHEW Policy on Protection of Human Subjects*. Washington, DC: U.S. Government Printing Office, 1971.
14. Curran, W.J. "The Approach of Two Federal Agencies." *Daedalus* 98 (1969):542-594.
15. *Institutional Guide to DHEW Policy on Protection of Human Subjects*.
16. National Research Act, P.L. 93-348, sections 201-205 (July 12, 1974).
17. 44 Fed. Reg. 47688 (1979).
18. 46 Fed. Reg. 8366 (1981).
19. Grundner, T.M. "DHHS Human Subjects Protection: The New Regulations Revisited." *Health Matrix* 1, no. 2 (1983): 37-41.
20. Grundner. "DHHS Human Subjects Protection."

Chapter 2

The Consent Process

The Importance of Consent

In the last chapter I talked briefly about some of the tragedies that prompted the development of governmental research regulation. Of these, none were more terrible than those revealed by the Nuremberg Tribunal following World War II. You may recall that one of the outcomes of this Tribunal was a set of basic principles called the Nuremberg Code and that virtually every major ethical code or set of human research guidelines developed since then have been based, at least in part, on these principles. Nowhere is this more true than in the area of informed consent. Indeed, it is the Nuremberg Code that provides us with the one overriding and inviolable principle of ethical research. It is of such importance, in fact, that if you learn nothing else from this book but this one principle, I will be quite pleased.

ANY RESEARCH PROJECT UTILIZING HUMAN SUBJECTS REQUIRES THE INFORMED CONSENT OF THOSE SUBJECTS [46.116].

No matter what the nature of the project, no matter how innocuous it may seem, no matter what you think one might be technically allowed to do according to governmental rulings, *the subjects have the right to know what they are getting into. They also have the right to say NO!* They have this right for good reason, for bad reason, or for no reason, and one of your main ethical responsibilities as a researcher is to insure that this right is honored. The principal vehicle for insuring it is the consent process.

There are a variety of ways of obtaining the consent of a subject, but almost all will involve some type of written documentation [46.117(a)].

Types of Consent Forms

There are two major ways of constructing a consent form, depending on how you plan to execute the consent. They are the short form and what we'll call the long form.

The *short form* is generally executed in three stages. First, in the presence of a witness, a very precisely worded oral presentation is made to the subject(s). This presentation should contain all the critical pieces of information that the subject(s) need to know to make an informed decision. Next, they are asked if they have any questions about the research or their role in it. After all questions have been answered, they are asked to sign a brief form stating, basically, that they have been given the information, that they understand what they are getting into, and that all their questions have been answered. This form is signed by each subject and the witness (you must have a witness, by the way, if you are going to use a short form). Finally, a written statement summarizing your oral presentation is signed by the witness and the person obtaining the consent, and a copy of this document along with a copy of the signed short form is given to each subject. You are then done.

The *long form* follows the same general procedures except that all necessary information is spelled out in the form that is signed. There is no summary sheet. In other words, the information that is presented orally to the subject in the short form now becomes the actual consent document in the long form. It, like the short form summary, is approved in advance by an IRB, read to (or by) the subject, and questions are requested. When the questions are answered, the subject signs two copies, keeps one, turns the other in to the researcher, and the process is complete.

While different researchers have different preferences as to which method they use, I'd like to put in a plug for the long form. To begin with, if you use the long form there is no question as to what was said or not said, promised or not promised to the subject. It's all there in black and white and it's signed. Second, the subject who can read what you are reading, while you are reading it, is more likely to understand what it was you said. He or she will not only understand it better, but his questions will be directed more toward clarifying his own thinking than understanding yours. Third, the subject will be able to keep a tangible signed copy of the consent agreement for future reference in case any question should arise in his mind as to the nature of the experiment, whom he should contact if any problems develop, etc. This, believe it or not, can become a positive factor in subject retention later on because planted in the consent form, among other things, is a list of all the advantages that are accruing to him (as well as to mankind and so forth) as a result of his participation in your noble project.

Obtaining Readability

A number of years ago when I was a graduate student, I took a job coordinating a very involved long-term research project with chronic alcoholics. Considering myself an ethically sensitive young researcher, one of the first things I did was to look over the consent forms being used. To my dismay, I found them deficient in a number of respects, so I rewrote them in long form and changed the consent process around.

More than a year later, while working with some formulas used by educators to determine the grade-level equivalence of reading material, I decided to test my consent forms. I was rather proud that my writing scored at the very highest levels--easily within graduate school range and easily capable of being included in the most scholarly of scholarly journals. My reaction, however, soon turned to horror when I realized that, in general, my subject population was lucky to have completed the seventh grade. By rewriting the forms, I had simultaneously made them both technically correct and totally unintelligible to the intended audience.

The moral of this story is probably obvious. *Always design your consent forms so they can be understood by your intended subject population* [46.116].

All people have a tendency to avoid asking questions that will betray their own areas of ignorance. The less educated they are, the less likely they will be to ask. Don't put your subjects in this position. Use a readability formula on your consent forms.

Now, exactly what are *readability formulas*? They are simple formulas you can use to determine the reading level of almost any written document. In most cases, they involve taking a few 100-word samples and counting up the number of sentences and/or syllables they contain. This information is then applied to a formula, and the outcome is the grade-level equivalency of the document.

It takes a while to go into all the details, so I am not going to try to do it here. However, I have included as an appendix a brief article on these formulas and how to use them (see Appendix B). Please take the time, either now or later, to read this article and apply it to your future work.

Procedures for Obtaining Consent

The process of obtaining consent is really quite simple. It's a three-step process to which we've already generally alluded.

Begin by gathering your subjects together either singly or in a group. Pass out two copies of the consent form to each of them and ask them to read along silently as you read it out loud. The reasons for this, by the way, are two-fold. First, it helps the subject to understand the material better if he can hear it as he reads. Secondly, and even more importantly, occasionally you will get a subject who can't read without glasses, or can't read well (with or without glasses). Sometimes the subject simply can't read at all and won't tell you! This is especially true if you are working with educationally-impaired or debilitated populations.

After having read it aloud, you may want to give a quick, informal verbal summary of what you have just read. This may not be necessary if, for example, you are working with college students. On the other hand, it may be very necessary if you are working with chronic alcoholics.

Although the regulations don't specifically require it, *always ask for questions when you have completed your presentation*. Be patient with these questions, encourage them, answer them fully, and above all, answer them truthfully.

Whatever you do, *never lie to a subject, or in any way force, coerce, or deceive him about what he is about to do*. This is supposed to be a "freely given, informed consent." It is *your* obligation to see that exactly that occurs.

There may be times when you can't tell the subject *everything* about a project because the design calls for deception. In other words, the subject must remain naive about the study's true intent if he or she is to give an honest reaction. Here again is an area that is not covered by the regulations and will require close cooperation between you and your IRB. In general, however, the way this is most often handled is by still conducting a consent session but leaving out (or deceiving the subject about) only those items that absolutely must be left out or altered in order to do the experiment. Then, after the subject is run, you must "debrief" the subject--revealing all--and seek his or her final consent. We will be saying more about this in Chapter 7.

In any event, when all questions have been answered, ask those who wish to be a part of the study to sign and date *both* copies of the consent form [46.117(a)]. It is important to remember here that *you must give the subject reasonable opportunity to consider whether or not to participate* [46.116].

This process is not to be a rushed affair. In general, the more the experiment exceeds "minimal risk" (see the definition in the introduction), the more the subject is expected to be given time for deliberation. If you are in doubt as to what constitutes a "reasonable opportunity," ask your local IRB chairperson for guidance.

Finally, collect one of the two completed consent forms from each of your subjects, explaining that the other is theirs to keep. Ideally, it is good if you can arrange to have a disinterested third party around who has observed the process.* He or she should sign the form where it says "Witness." The consent execution is now complete. You may give the subjects further instructions as to what to do next, when to appear, etc.

---

* If you are using a "short form," the presence of a witness is mandatory [46.117(b)(2)].

As you can see, the general framework for obtaining consent is not very complicated. In general, you need to design a form (preferably the long form) that is complete yet understandable to the subjects. You read them the forms, answer any questions, give them a reasonable amount of time to deliberate, and have those who wish to participate sign up.

Verbal Consent and No Consent at All

It is understood that there are times when a verbal-only consent is all that can be obtained. It is also understood that these exceptions are relatively few and far between. If you must do it that way, be sure you have double-checked this conclusion with your Institutional Review Board and be sure you've read Chapter 7 about altering or waiving the consent process.

Finally, if you feel you simply cannot bring yourself to do a consent *at all*, that's fine too. But at the same time, you might also want to consider some of the many exciting challenges that are offered in the world of animal experimentation.

I am serious. Conducting research using human subjects without having any form of consent at all is, in my view, indefensible.

Now, I realize that I have not mentioned anything yet about exactly what is supposed to go into the forms. We are going to get into that in the next chapter. But first, let's try a few simple situations covering what we've learned so far.

Turn to page 17.

Situation 1

Oddisee Wentworth is a graduate student of yours who is doing his dissertation on short-term recall. The project calls for the subject merely to respond to a set of nonsense syllables presented on a microcomputer. You ask him about his informed consent plans.

Oddisee explains that because the project involves no physical or mental risk to anyone (except perhaps to Oddisee who has the task of getting the computer program to work properly) and because, fortunately, he has a number of subjects "temporarily available" in his Introductory Psychology class this semester, he has decided to proceed without using any sort of consent process at all. After all, it's only a small project, he is only a graduate student, no risk is involved to the subject, and he needs every last subject he can get his hands on.

Is Oddisee justified in not using a consent process?

Yes. Turn to page 19.

No. Turn to page 20.

You said, "Yes, Oddisee is justified in not using a consent process." You also answered INCORRECTLY.

If you recall, I said a few pages back, "ANY RESEARCH PROJECT UTILIZING HUMAN SUBJECTS REQUIRES THE CONSENT OF THOSE SUBJECTS." The fact that there is no foreseeable risk (in Oddisee's eyes anyway) does not enter into it. You must allow the subject to decide that for himself.

The fact that it is only a small project or that Oddisee is still a graduate student, is also irrelevant. No matter what size the project is, if human beings are involved, the project requires the consent of those humans. Finally, the worst reason of all is that there is a "temporarily available" subject pool around upon which to do your research. This reason implies a lack of sensitivity to the right each person has to be treated in accordance with established ethical principles while serving as a subject in experimentation.

Reread the section of the chapter opening entitled "The Importance of Consent" as well as my little diatribe under the section titled "Verbal Consent and No Consent at All." **Then continue to page 21.**

You said, "No, Oddisee is not justified in ignoring the consent process." You answered CORRECTLY.

Obviously, your keen, discerning eye noted the statement above that said, "ANY RESEARCH PROJECT UTILIZING HUMAN SUBJECTS REQUIRES THE CONSENT OF THOSE SUBJECTS." You understood that the size of the project, Oddisee's student status, the degree of risk, and the availability of the subject population were irrelevant to the fact that subjects have certain rights that must be explained and protected, and that the consent process is the best way of doing this.

Nice work. **Continue to page 21.**

Situation 2

Professor Eager is newly arrived at West Overshoe Tech. It is his first assignment at a "big name" school and he is anxious to prove himself to the older faculty and students. To obtain this approval, not to mention tenure, he must publish. Because you like the cut of his Van Dyke beard, you volunteer to be his graduate assistant.

He wants to run a sociological research project on high school dropouts and has published a call for volunteers in the local newspapers. He gives you a copy of the consent form to be used and you look it over, noting with approval that it contains all the necessary items. However, you are suspicious of the wording of it.

You remember an article in Appendix B of a wonderful textbook you once read about using readability formulas on consent forms, so you look it up, apply it, and sure enough, the form tests out at a graduate school reading level. You are on your way to Professor Eager's office to tell him his consent form is not valid when you stop to inform your roommate of what you are about to do.

He urges you to forget about it. Why jeopardize your degree by making some professor mad? Who are you to say it's not valid? Besides, you're just assisting. Eager has the responsibility, not you.

Do you continue to Professor Eager's office or not?

Yes. Turn to page 23.

No. Turn to page 25.

You are absolutely CORRECT.

No doubt you have concluded that the responsibility for ethical research falls on *everyone's* shoulders. It is not solely the responsibility of the institution, the Institutional Review Board, the principal investigator, or the technician. All have equal and parallel obligations.

You must also have concluded that there is no way a consent can be "informed" if the consent form itself is unintelligible to the subject. On this ground alone, Professor Eager's consent form was invalid, and you had every right (and every obligation) to tell him so.

Very good. **Continue to page 29.**

You are WRONG.

To begin with, ethical research is *everyone's* responsibility. The obligation to see that a truly informed consent occurs is not solely that of the institution, the review board, the principal investigator, or the technician. Everyone has a co-equal and parallel obligation to see that it occurs.

In addition, there is no way that a consent can be "informed" if the form itself is unintelligible to the subject. On this ground alone, Professor Eager's consent was invalid and you had every right (not to mention obligation) to tell him so.

Reread the section "Obtaining Readability," then **continue on to page 29.**

HEY, WHY ARE YOU READING THIS PAGE?

Nowhere are you directed here. You are either reading the pages in between the ones you are supposed to be on, or you are confused as to what to do.

If it is the former, have fun. It will take you longer to work through the program but you might pick up some additional information.

If it is the latter and you are confused, go back to the "To the Reader" page (after the introduction) and refresh your memory as to how this book is to be used.

Situation 3

A colleague from the Department of Medicine has asked you to sit in as a witness to the consent process for a moderately high risk study he wants to do.

You've looked at his consent forms earlier and they are in good shape. They are complete and readable. He assembled his first group of potential subjects in one of the hospital's small auditoriums and distributed two copies of the form to each of them. He then read the form out loud while each subject read along silently. Finally, he asked all those who were interested in participating in the project to sign and date the form at the bottom and pass one copy back to him--they could keep the other copy for their records. All those not wishing to participate were asked to pass both their forms in, were dismissed in a friendly fashion, and thanked for their time.

While the remaining group was signing and dating their forms, he walks over to you and asks whether he forgot anything.

Did he forget anything?

Yes. Turn to page 31.
No. Turn to page 33.

You are RIGHT.

You noticed that he forgot two very important things. First, he forgot to ask the subjects whether they had any questions. Second, he gave the subjects absolutely no time to consider participation.

Congratulations on picking these items up.

Please continue to page 35.

You are WRONG.

He committed two errors. First, he did not allow for any sort of question and answer interchange. Second, there was no time allowed for the subjects to deliberate on what they had been told.

You have to keep in mind that some people are more forthright about questions than others. Some people wouldn't hesitate to interrupt things to ask a question. Other people are more reluctant; they sometimes need to be prodded a bit, or at the least, given a clear opportunity to ask. You must provide this opportunity.

You also must provide some sort of opportunity for the subjects to think about what you have just outlined. In the case of minimal risk studies, this need not necessarily be a huge quantity of time, but there should at least be some sort of break between the questions and answers and the actual signing.

Reread the section "Procedures for Obtaining Consent," and **continue to page 35.**

Situation 4

Part of your responsibilities as Director of Nursing at a major hospital is to encourage the development of nursing research. As an experienced researcher yourself, you are glad to do so, and several staff members have already come to you for assistance.

You are in the last stages of helping one of your newer, but most promising, nurses shape up her research protocol. Everything seems to be ready to go, but you haven't yet looked at her consent plans. You ask for the consent form and ask her how she plans to execute it.

First, you look over the form itself. It seems to have all the necessary items and, according to the readability check, it is well within the range of her proposed population.

Her consent process is as follows: She plans to gather her subjects together in one group, pass out two copies of the consent form and read it aloud to them as they silently read along. Following this, she will give a quick verbal summary in informal language and ask for any questions. After all questions have been answered she will show the subjects the equipment to be used or show them around the facility--anything to provide a break in the proceedings--and allow the subjects time to make up their minds. When this is done, she will ask those who wish to participate to sign and date both copies of the form. One copy will be passed in and the other will be kept by the subjects for their own records. Finally, she will have the witness countersign each form while she collects the extras from those who chose not to participate and dismisses them in a friendly fashion. When this is over, she will give further instructions to those who remain.

Has she indeed set up her consent process properly?

Yes, she has. Turn to page 37.
No, she has not. Turn to page 38.

You said, "Yes, she has." You are CORRECT!

You remembered all the details of the consent process: readability, two copies of the form, reading the form out loud, asking for questions, a question and answer period, break, signing and dating both copies and, as an option, having a witness.

Very good! Let's move on to the next section where we will learn how to design the consent form itself.

Turn to page 39.

You said, "No, she hasn't." You are WRONG.

Why hasn't she? She included all the necessary steps. Her form was in the proper readability range for her particular subject population, she provided two copies of the form, she read the form out loud, asked for questions, held a break, and had them sign and date both copies. She even had a witness to the event which, with a long form, is optional. What more do you want?

If you are still confused at this point as to how the consent process should function, reread the section "Procedures for Obtaining Consent," and work through Situations 1 to 4 again.

When you are ready, **continue on page 39.**

Chapter 3

Consent Form Content: The Beginning Section

The Consent Form

You now know that (1) you must use a consent form, (2) it must be understandable to your subjects and, (3) the steps involved in the process of obtaining consent. But you still don't know exactly what is supposed to go into the consent form itself. That is what we are going to take up now.

All good consent forms (like love stories, movie scripts, and graduate programs) have a beginning, a middle, and an end. Each section has certain pieces of information that must be contained in it. Below is the full list. Look them over before we start examining them one at a time.

Beginning Section

1. Who is doing the experiment.
2. The nature, purpose, and duration of the experiment--including the fact that the procedure is experimental.
3. The uses to be made of the data.

Middle Section

1. The methods to be employed.
2. The hazards, inconveniences, and risks the subject will undergo, so far as they are known.
3. The availability of compensation and treatment, if injured.
4. The benefits that might be expected.
5. Disclosure of alternate procedures the subject may choose if the experiment is therapeutically related.
6. The conditions of participation, if any.

End Section

1. A statement of the extent to which the data is confidential and a description of the procedures to be employed in maintaining that confidentiality.
2. The fact that the subject is at liberty to withdraw his prior consent to the experiment or discontinue participation in the experiment at any time without prejudice.
3. An offer to answer any questions and instructions as to how to contact someone should questions arise later.
4. A place for the date of signing and for the signature of the subject and witness.
5. And finally, a procedural reminder that there can be no exculpatory language anywhere in the form.

Let's start at the beginning.

The Beginning Section

The opening section of a consent form should contain three pieces of information:

1. Who is doing the experiment.
2. The nature, purpose, and duration of the experiment--including the fact that the procedure is experimental.
3. The uses to be made of the data.

The consent form should begin by letting the subject know *who is doing the experiment*. While this may seem obvious, it is frequently overlooked and it is important for at least three reasons.

First, it can be a very important factor in the subject's decision whether or not to participate in the project at all. Research being run by the National Institutes of Health or Harvard University may be one thing; a project being done by the American Nazi Party or some "anti-war" group may be quite another.

Second, it lets the subjects know who to contact six months from now if they wake up at 3:00 A.M. covered with shaggy red hair and protruding incisor teeth. In other words, it is a vehicle for accountability.

Finally, it's a nice way to start off the form. It's like saying, "Hi there, my name is . . . " only in this case you would say something like, "The Institute for Counseling Services is carrying out research into various ways of controlling anxiety."

A second and equally important element of the consent form is a *statement of the nature, purpose, and duration of the experiment--including the fact that the procedure is experimental* [46.116(a)(1)]. Here, again, is some very important information if the subject is to make an intelligent, "informed" decision as to whether or not to participate. While, at this point, the statement does not have to be extensive, it should be accurate and should contain some indication of previous work done in the area. Something such as the following should suffice:

> We are attempting to determine whether a new biofeedback procedure will work in relieving test anxiety in college freshmen. While we know this procedure is effective with underachieving high school students, it has never been tried with college-age students. Your role in the project will consist of attending six one-hour experimental sessions spaced approximately one week apart.

The third element of the consent form details the *uses to be made of the data*. For example, a project designed to collect IQ data to demonstrate the inherent inferiority of a particular race may find objecting subjects. Once again, the statement need not be extensive. A simple, "eventually these data will be used to improve the counseling program at West Overshoe Tech" will do.

If you have not already pieced together the above three examples, let's do so now. A good opening to a consent form, then, might look like this:

> The Institute for Counseling Services is carrying out research into various ways of controlling anxiety. We are attempting to determine whether a new biofeedback procedure will work in relieving test anxiety in college freshmen. While we know this procedure is effective with underachieving high school students, it has never been tried with college-age students. Your role in the project will consist of attending six one-hour experimental sessions spaced approximately one week apart. Eventually these data will be used to improve the counseling program at West Overshoe Tech.

Presto! Only 89 words and you are already a third of the way through the form.

Let's try a few more examples of the consent form opening.

Situation 5

A student of yours is writing her dissertation on the effect of a particular self-punishment procedure on smoking behavior. She shows you her consent form. It begins as follows:

> As part of a dissertation project in the Department of Psychology at West Overshoe Tech, an inquiry is being conducted into the effectiveness of a particular self-control technique on smoking. Basically we are attempting to find out whether this procedure, known as "coverent control," can be used to stop or reduce smoking in adult males. While it has been shown effective in weight control and drinking behavior, no attempt has been made to use it with smokers. Data from this study may be published, but at no time will your name be used.

Is this an appropriate beginning for her consent form?

Yes. Turn to page 45.

No. Turn to page 46.

You said, "Yes, it is an appropriate beginning." You are WRONG.

The opening failed to state the expected duration of the experiment. Will the subject be involved in this enterprise a few hours, a week, a month, or for the rest of his life? It could well make a difference to your subject (or anyone else for that matter).

Remember, the consent form must contain the nature, purpose, and *duration* of the experiment.

Turn to page 47.

You said, "No, it is not an appropriate beginning."
You are absolutely CORRECT!

The opening contains statements of who is doing the experiment, the uses to be made of the data, its nature, and its purpose; however, it does not make any mention of the *duration* of the experiment. Obviously, the experiment's duration could well be a major factor in whether an individual would choose to be a part of it or not.

Nice work!!

Continue to page 47.

Situation 6

As a young, first-year physiology professor, you are invited to witness a consent session being done by your departmental chairperson. You arrive a few minutes early and look over the consent form. It begins as follows:

> We are conducting a study to learn about the influence of Vitamin A on an individual's ability to perceive objects. It will require you to appear at a single one-hour experimental session. No experimental procedures will be employed beyond this one visit. This information, along with other data we are gathering, will be useful in analyzing the extent to which this substance can be used to enhance the alertness and perceptual abilities of pilots and other skilled equipment operators.

Is this a proper opening?

Yes. Turn to page 49.

No. Turn to page 50.

You said, "Yes, it is a proper opening." You are WRONG.

Who is the "we" conducting the experiment? Is it prestigious West Overshoe Tech or the National Association for the Establishment of Thought Control? Would it make a difference to you which it was? Then why wouldn't it make a difference to your subjects? Identify yourself or your organization explicitly. (No, Xeroxing the consent form on your letterhead doesn't count.)

Reread the section entitled, "The Beginning Section" as it pertains to identifying who is doing the experiment.

When you are ready, **turn to page 51.**

You said, "No, it is not a proper opening." You are RIGHT!

Obviously, you noticed that the "we" that is doing the survey is never identified. Obviously you also know that the subject needs to know this in order to make an informed decision. Very good.

Go on to page 51.

Situation 7

A postdoctoral fellow arrives at your hospital fresh from residency training. Having come from a far less enlightened program than yours, he has not had the benefit of this instructional unit. He designs a consent form for a small project he wants to run and, because you are a member of the hospital IRB, he shows it to you for your comment. The complete form reads as follows:

> I have been informed of the purpose and procedures involved in the study of the relationship between stress and dyspepsia, and I am a voluntary participant. I understand that I may withdraw this consent at any time.

Is it all right?

Yes. Turn to page 53.

No. Turn to page 54.

You answered, "Yes, it's all right."

Come on! This "consent" bears no resemblance to what is necessary for a valid form. It not only has a bad beginning, it has an impossible middle and an outrageous end (and we haven't even talked about *that* yet).

Reread the chapter opening. Then go back to Situation 7 and choose the other answer. You might find some information there that will surprise you.

You said, "No, it is not all right."
CORRECT.

This mess bears no resemblance to a consent form. Interestingly enough, however, with the exception of changing the subject of the research, this is an actual consent form that was used on a major project. To make things even worse, it had been approved by an Institutional Review Board!

Shake your head ruefully, and **turn to page 55**.

Situation 8

One of your nursing graduate students is about to submit her thesis proposal to your school's Human Subjects Committee. She calls you up and says she's worried about possible delays. She wants to make sure everything is correct so it will go through smoothly.

You meet over coffee in the hospital cafeteria, chat sympathetically with her for a while on the irrationality of some of the course requirements, and finally get down to business. The opening paragraph of her consent form reads as follows:

> As part of a master's thesis in the Department of Nursing at West Overshoe Tech, I am attempting to determine the effectiveness of a new programmed text in nursing research ethics. While programmed texts have been in existence for many years, their effectiveness in teaching ethics has remained unclear. To date, only one limited dissertation project has been attempted in this area. Your role will be to participate in one afternoon session of approximately three hours' duration and, at a later date, to allow inspection of your final thesis or dissertation proposal. The purpose of this research is to refine the programmed materials for possible later adoption by the department. No further use of this data will be made.

What do you think? Did she get it right?

Yes. Turn to page 57.

No. Turn to page 58.

You said, "Yes, she did get it right."
You are also RIGHT.

She included all the information necessary for a valid opening paragraph. She mentioned who is doing the work, its nature, purpose, and duration, and what uses will be made of the data.

Excellent. Now let's get into the middle portion of the consent form.

Turn to page 59.

You said, "No, she did not get it right."
You are WRONG.

What more are you looking for? She included all the information necessary for a valid opening paragraph. She mentioned who is doing the work, its nature, purpose, duration, and what uses will be made of the data.

If you are still confused at this point as to what should be in the opening section, go back and reread the chapter opening and work through Situations 5 through 8 again. Then turn to page 59.

If you are not confused but still got it wrong--try to figure out why you thought it was wrong and reread the relevant portions of the chapter opening. Upon completion, go get a cup of coffee.

When you get back, **turn to page 59.**

Chapter 4

Consent Form Content: The Middle Section

The middle section of a consent form must contain at least three and possibly as many as six pieces of information. Whether you use more than three will depend on the kind of research you are doing and its relative risk. Let's start by looking at the six possible items and reviewing each in turn.

1. The methods to be employed.
2. The hazards, inconveniences, and risks the subject will undergo, so far as they are known.
3. The availability of compensation and treatment, if injured.
4. The benefits that might be expected from participating in the project.
5. Disclosure of alternate procedures the subject may choose if the experiment is therapeutically related.
6. The conditions of participation, if any.

In general, the middle section is probably the most difficult to write. The problem, simply put, is this: You must put down enough information for the subject to make an intelligent and informed decision--but not so much, or so technically, that he or she gets mixed up. You are walking a tightrope between full disclosure and total confusion; it is not an easy task.

From an ethical standpoint, it would be ideal if all research were conducted only on M.D.'s or Ph.D.'s. Preferably, these would be people in the same discipline as the one in which you are conducting research, and even more preferably, people who specialize in the specific issue with which you are dealing. There would be little question then that the subjects would fully understand what they are getting into.

As fascinating as the prospect may seem, you are not (in most cases anyway) dealing with colleagues as subjects. You are dealing most of the time with people who are totally unfamiliar with your field of study and the research you are about to undertake. Your explanation is critical. It must be accurate, complete, and above all, *simple*. The task is not as hopeless as it might seem, however, if you just use a little common sense.

For example, when you finish writing the middle section of your form (or any part of the form for that matter), do the obvious--try it out on someone. Snatch someone out of the student union, ask a secretary, or look for someone waiting at a bus stop if you have to. (Roommates and relatives work especially well for this sort of thing.) Give them a copy of the text. Ask them if they understand it. Have them explain it back to you in their own words. Does it come back garbled or accurate? Ask them some questions about it to see if they understand. Believe me, if your version is confusing, you'll learn about it very quickly this way.

One of the first items to be included in the middle section is a statement of *the methods to be employed* [46.116(a)(1)]. By this we do not mean the methods to be employed by *you*. We are not interested in the type of statistical analysis you're going to use. The subjects couldn't care less. We want to know what, *from the subject's standpoint,* he or she is going to be expected to do. Something, perhaps, like this:

> At these experimental sessions you will be introduced to a biofeedback relaxation procedure by a staff member who is experienced in this technique. The session itself consists of learning to relax by using a device that tells you how tense or relaxed your muscles are. When the device is connected, it will make clicking sounds. Your job will be to sit back, relax, and by relaxing, try to make the clicking sounds decrease in frequency.

The second thing that needs to be included is one of the most important elements in the entire consent form: *a statement of the hazards, discomforts, or risks the subject will undergo, so far as they are known* [46.116(a)(2)]. Here again is another "fine line." You need to be honest and accurate without, at the same time, being ridiculous. A statement like: "The possibility exists that you might trip coming up the steps of the laboratory" is not quite what we have in mind.

If there are risks or discomforts that may potentially occur in the experiment, even if they are of fairly low probability, you must state them. For example: "Some subjects have found listening to 'white noise' for extended periods of time to be somewhat uncomfortable. Others (less than 5%) have reported slightly reduced hearing abilities for a period of up to one hour after the experimental session. However, no instances of impaired hearing beyond this one-hour point have ever been reported."

While we're on the subject of risk, if there is any likelihood that a subject could be hurt, i.e., more than "minimal risk," the regulations require that *you must report on the availability of compensation and treatment should the subject be injured* [46.116(a)(6)]. If you cannot offer any compensation or free treatment, then you must say that too. In any event, play it safe. If you are in doubt as to whether this clause should be in your consent form, ask your local IRB chairperson. He or she will be glad to give you a ruling on it.

Many experiments within the behavioral sciences, of course, carry no realistic risk of physical or mental harm. Even so, you must remember that your subjects do not necessarily know this. You should still make a negative report, something like: "There are no risks or discomforts connected with this procedure." Just be sure you don't jump too quickly. You may want to consider using this rule of thumb: *If the experiment exposes the subject to risks greater than what might be expected during the course of a normal day, state it.*

The next item in this section of the consent form is one that is frequently omitted. What makes this particularly unusual is the fact that it is an item that, in terms of subject recruitment, works in the researcher's favor. This is supposed to be an informed consent, right? It is supposed to help the subject decide whether or not to participate, right? Weigh the good and the bad, the positive and the negative? Well, if you are going to tell your subjects all the grim news about risks and hazards, how about telling them some of the good stuff as well: *the potential benefits that might be expected from participating in the project* [46.116(a)(3)]. Don't be modest! If you have reason to believe they are likely to benefit personally from the procedure, then tell them something like, "We have reason to believe that this procedure may be of help in the treatment of ... "

If no direct personal benefit is likely to occur, you can always cite the possible benefits accruing to mankind. For example, "While no direct benefit is likely to accrue to yourself as a result of your participation, you may well have the pride of knowing that you have contributed to a major research effort to help ... "

If your project is neither of benefit to the subject nor, at least theoretically, of benefit to mankind--why are you doing it?

The next item (stay with me just a little while longer) is a special case of conducting a research project for a therapeutic purpose. In this situation, you have a subject who is either undergoing another form of treatment or potentially could undergo another form of treatment than the one you are offering him. If this is the case, *you must disclose to the subject what those alternatives are* [46.116(a)(4)]. This does not need to be extensive: "Should you decide not to participate in this project, you will still be eligible for all the regular counseling services" will do.

Finally, *if you have any conditions of participation, you must disclose them* [46.116(b)(4)]. In other words, if the subject must participate in your research to receive some benefit, or if you have some condition attached to participation, such as the subject must agree to stay in the research project for at least six months, then you must disclose it. We'll be saying more about this in Chapter 6.

Okay, so once more, let's piece together the examples we've given so far in this section. A fairly typical middle section, then, might look something like this:

> At these experimental sessions you will be introduced to a biofeedback relaxation procedure by a staff member who is experienced in this technique. The session itself consists of learning to relax by using a device that tells you how tense or relaxed your muscles are. When the device is connected, it will make clicking sounds. Your job is to sit back, relax, and by relaxing, try to make the clicking sounds decrease in frequency. There are no known risks or discomforts associated with this procedure. We have reason to believe that this method may be of significant value in treating test anxiety. However, should you decide not to participate in this project, you will still be eligible for all the regular counseling services.

Situation 9

Oddisee is finally straightened out on the consent form for his short-term recall experiment (remember Situation 1?). He decided to have a consent process after all. The opening of his consent form was fine. The middle section read like this:

> Should you decide to participate in this project you will be expected to attend three half-hour sessions in the course of a 10-day period. Upon arrival at the laboratory, a staff member will explain the procedures you are to follow. There are no known risks or inconveniences associated with this experiment, and the knowledge we gain may be of substantial value in the future design of curricular materials.

Is the middle section of his form right?

Yes. Turn to page 65.

No. Turn to page 66.

You said, "Yes, the middle section of his consent form is all right."
You are WRONG.

Oddisee never explains to the people exactly what it is they are expected to do when they become subjects. The phrase, "Upon arrival at the laboratory, a staff member will explain the procedures you are to follow" will not do. It is far too vague.

Reread the paragraph on "methods to be employed," and **go to page 67**.

You said, "No, the middle section of this consent form is not all right."
Absolutely CORRECT!

No doubt you noticed that Oddisee never explains what it is the subject is supposed to do. The subject, of course, must know this if he is to make an informed choice.

Nice work!

Continue to page 67.

Situation 10

Your departmental chairperson is doing a study of the effects of concentrated Vitamin A on perceptual abilities. The vitamin is perfectly harmless in the quantities to be used in his study. You've straightened out the problems she had with the opening. Now she comes back to you (you are becoming the departmental expert on research ethics) with the following middle section:

> You will be given a pill containing a small quantity of Vitamin A and, 15 minutes later, will be shown a panel of lights with a series of switches in front of it. You will be asked to turn on certain switches based on which lights you see flash in front of you. At the end of this period you will undergo an interview about your experience which should last no more than 15 minutes. After this interview, you will be paid $10.00 for helping in this study.

Did she do it right?

Yes. Turn to page 69.
No. Turn to page 70.

You said, "Yes, the middle section of the consent form was complete."
You are WRONG.

I know it might be easy to overlook something like a negative report, but you've got to say it anyway: "There are no known risks or discomforts to be expected in participating in this study" or words to that effect.

I can see how you might miss it, but it really needs to be there.

Turn to page 71.

You said, "No, the middle section of the consent form is not complete."
Absolutely CORRECT!
Very good.

You obviously realized that this section was missing a statement on risk and discomforts. A lot of people would have overlooked this item for the simple reason that there were no risks. You remembered that all forms must have it, even if it is a negative report.

Onward to page 71.

Situation 11

You have been appointed to the IRB at the big state mental hospital in West Overshoe. To familiarize yourself with the committee's operations you decide to look through some of their files.

You come across a study which attempted to evaluate a new psychotherapeutic procedure for reducing stress in patients being treated for high anxiety conditions. The middle section of the consent form read as follows:

> Your participation will consist of a one-visit physical evaluation by a staff physician followed by a series of 10 clinical treatments. Each treatment will last one hour and will occur twice a week for five weeks. The physical evaluation will consist of the measurement of your pulse and blood pressure. The clinical treatments will consist of conversation with a therapist. Neither procedure involves any known physical risk or discomfort, although the conversation may be about things or situations that some people find upsetting. During the clinical treatments, you will be asked to complete several checklists regarding your emotional state.
>
> We believe that this new procedure shows great promise for being helpful for your present condition and that your participation may lead to further refinements that will help others with conditions similar to yours.

Is this middle section complete?

Yes. Turn to page 73.

No. Turn to page 74.

Your answer is WRONG.

Remember, this study is being conducted at a state mental hospital. Everyone there is presumably undergoing a therapeutic regimen of some sort. If you are going to introduce an experimental procedure, you have to disclose what alternative procedures are available, including continuation of their present therapy.

Reread the paragraph stating, "You must disclose to the subject what those alternatives are."

Continue to page 75.

You said, "No, this middle section is not complete."

Your answer is CORRECT.

Undoubtedly, you noticed that the study was being conducted in a state mental hospital. Further, you remembered that when you introduce an experimental procedure in this type of setting, you must also present the alternative therapies that are available.

Good work!

Turn to page 75.

Situation 12

You are sitting in the hospital cafeteria with one of your nursing graduate students again, amiably watching your coffee get cold. The opening paragraph of her consent form was okay, but now you have gotten to the middle section. It reads:

> At this afternoon session, you will be given a pre-test on your knowledge of research ethics and will be given a series of programmed materials. You will work through these materials and, upon completion, will be given a post-test. The entire process will take about one hour. At a later date, when you have developed an approved thesis or dissertation proposal, it will be examined by a member of this research team for its ethical integrity and compared with the proposals of others who have not been exposed to these materials. There are, of course, no known hazards, inconveniences, or risks associated with this procedure other than, perhaps, the inconvenience of having donated an afternoon of your time. On the other hand, you may well take some pride in participating in an effort to increase the ethical educational level of the profession you have chosen to enter.

Is it okay?

Yes. Turn to page 77.
No. Turn to page 78.

You said, "Yes, she did make an error."
You are WRONG!

Where did she make an error? She included a statement of the methods to be employed, the hazards, inconveniences, risks, and any benefits to be expected. A statement of alternate procedures, of course, is not required because this is not a therapeutic situation. The availability of compensation and treatment is not mentioned because the realistic probability of harm is nil. And, the conditions of participation are not mentioned because the subject's participation is unconditional.

Reread any parts of the chapter opening that you may be confused about.

When you are ready, **turn to page 79.**

You said, "No, she did not make an error."
You are CORRECT.

She included a statement of the methods to be employed, any hazards, inconveniences, or risks, and any benefits to be expected. You also noticed that a statement of alternate procedures, compensation, and conditions of participation were not needed in this case.

Very good.

Turn to page 79.

Situation 13

Just down the road from the campus of West Overshoe Tech is a very prestigious private research firm called "Overshoe Research, Inc." Recently they landed a contract from a large manufacturing concern to establish the effectiveness of a series of newspaper ads the company is planning to run. To do this, they will be securing a number of volunteer subjects and testing their reactions to the ads. Each volunteer will be paid $3.50 per hour for their time.

As a faculty member in West Overshoe's high-powered Department of Psychology, you have been called in as a consultant on this project. During the course of your work, you come across a copy of the consent form they will use. Its middle section reads like this:

> During the experimental session, you will be asked to look through an eyepiece into a machine that will display various advertisements on a screen. Each picture will remain visible for about 10 seconds. While the picture is visible, the machine will measure whether the size of the pupillary openings in your eyes has increased or decreased. This procedure is absolutely painless and there are no known hazards, risks, or inconveniences associated with it.

Is there something missing?

Yes. Turn to page 81.
No. Turn to page 83.

You said, "Yes, there is something missing."

You are absolutely right.

Very good. You picked up on the fact that, although the subjects were being paid $3.50 an hour to participate, no mention was made of it in the consent form. That constitutes a benefit which should be mentioned.

Nice job!

Go to page 85.

You said, "No, there is nothing missing."
WRONG.

Remember, early in the description of the situation it was mentioned that each subject would receive $3.50 per hour for their time. That constitutes a benefit and should be reported in the form. I mean, why hide it? It's a legitimate benefit and should be presented to the subject, along with the other information, as part of his or her consideration.

If you are confused about the benefit issue, reread the paragraphs on "the potential benefits that might be expected from participating in the project."

Go to page 85.

Situation 14

A sociology student, who has been assigned this same textbook, has tried his hand at doing a hypothetical consent form. He shows you the result of his attempt at writing the first two sections. It reads as follows:

> The Institute for Behavioral Science, in conjunction with the West Overshoe Public Library, is carrying out a survey of leisure time activities and reading habits. While studies of college students have been done, no attempt has yet been made to survey the general public in this regard. The results of this study will be used to help determine the purchasing pattern of the West Overshoe Public Library for the next year.
>
> If you choose to participate, you will be asked to keep track of the amount of free time you have and the materials (books, magazines, newspapers, etc.) that you read over the next 30 days. There are, of course, no hazards or risks involved in such activity and you will be inconvenienced only so far as the time it takes to keep the necessary records. We expect these data will help the public library to meet your reading needs and the needs of the rest of the community even better in the future.

What do you think? Is it adequate?

Yes. Turn to page 87.
No. Turn to page 89.

You said, "Yes, it is adequate."
And indeed it is.
It meets all the requirements for both the beginning and the middle sections.
Congratulations, you remembered all the way back to the beginning.

Turn to page 91.

You said, "No, it is not adequate."
You are WRONG.

Why isn't it adequate? It tells us who is doing the experiment, the nature, purpose, and duration of the experiment--including the fact that it is a "first." It tells the method to be used, the hazards, inconveniences, and the risks to be expected, as well as the benefits.

So what more do you want?

If your problem was with the first paragraph, reread the opening of Chapter 3.

If your problem was with the second paragraph, reread the opening of Chapter 4.

If you had problems with both, then reread them both.

When you are finished, **go to page 91.**

Chapter 5

Consent Form Content: The Ending

So now that we've gotten the beginning and the middle sections put together, we come at last to the final touches of the consent form.

The beginning section was an introduction. It generally served to put the subject on notice as to what the project was all about. The middle section was a more detailed description of the project's methodology, what the researcher expected of the subject, and what the subject could expect from the research. The end section, however, is really a list of two guarantees and three procedural reminders. They are as follows:

1. A statement that the data are confidential and a description of the procedures to be employed in maintaining that confidentiality.
2. The fact that the subject is at liberty to withdraw his consent prior to the experiment, or discontinue participation in the experiment at any time, without prejudice.
3. An offer to answer any questions as well as instructions as to how to contact someone should questions arise later.
4. A place for the date of signing and for the signature of the subject and witness.
5. And finally, a procedural reminder that there can be no exculpatory language anywhere in the form.

Again, let's take them one at a time.

The first guarantee is a statement that *the data are confidential, and gives a description of the procedures to be employed to maintain that confidentiality* [46.116(a)(5)].

Look at it this way. Your interest in doing the experiment is not to find out how John Doe, *as John Doe,* reacts to a particular experiment. Your interest is in finding out how John Doe as Subject 78-324 reacts. Names and identities are normally irrelevant to your work. You must guarantee and protect the confidentiality of your data. This is especially true when the data being gathered are of an intimate, illegal, or potentially embarrassing nature. For most situations, you could say something like: "All information will remain strictly confidential. Although the findings of this study may be published, at no time will your name be used."

For studies dealing with more sensitive information, however, you may want to go into a more elaborate statement; for example, "All information will remain strictly confidential. The data you give us will be maintained in a locked file cabinet and organized by code number. The name key for that code will be kept locked in a separate location" (or whatever your procedures are).

There is another related area that you need to know something about because someday it could become very important to both you and your subjects. I am speaking here about the area of "privilege." As you are probably aware, information gathered in the course of a therapy session or medical interview is considered "privileged information." In other words, it is confidential information between the therapist or physician and the patient, and no court can force anyone to reveal anything of its nature. Information gathered in the course of a research project, however, *does not* come under this classification. You could, at least theoretically, be called into court and forced to divulge what you know about a subject. *You must keep this in mind if you are doing research in a legally sensitive area.*

There are basically four general ways of dealing with this legal incongruity. First, you can avoid the problem by not using subject names on anything--including the consent forms. If there are no names on the data and the individual subjects are not identifiable, and if there are no names on the consent forms, there is nothing to worry about. This is the easiest solution, and we will be talking more about how to obtain this kind of consent form waiver in Chapter 7. Unfortunately, it is not always possible to do this. You may want to do a follow-up on your subjects, for example, in which you want to compare their first set of responses to their second. To do that, you need to know which data belongs to whom.

A second possibility is to notify your subjects up front that, while you will do your best to protect the confidentiality of the data, you could legally be called into court and the research records subpoenaed.

Third, you could attempt to avoid a court order by coding the data and putting the key to the code in an inaccessible place. For example, a friend of mine was doing a research project of a legally sensitive nature in Detroit, Michigan. He kept track of his subjects with code numbers. The key to the code was kept in a strong box across the river in Windsor, Canada. To gain access to the subject code, authorities would have to process the subpoena through the Canadian government via the U.S. State Department and would involve negotiations literally at an ambassadorial level. Not many agencies would be willing to run that kind of bureaucratic gauntlet. He was liable for contempt of court charges, but the data were relatively safe.

Finally, you could simply refuse any court order and take your chances.

I am *not* advising you to adopt either of these last two courses of action. Both are, at present at least, illegal, but they *are* options. In the meantime, the only thing you can do is hope you never get into that position, and support efforts to change the law so that research data does become privileged information.

The second item of the final section is easily the most important statement in the entire form. In my opinion, if you don't have it, your consent form is worthless! Period! *The subject is at liberty to withdraw his or her consent and discontinue participation at any time without prejudice* [46.116(a)(8)]. If consent means anything at all, it means that the subject has the right to say "NO!" He has that right before he signs the consent form, he has the right after he signs the consent form, he has the right up to the last second of the last session of the last experiment you will ever run. It is inalienable and absolute, and there are no circumstances in which you can arbitrarily remove that right from him or pressure or deceive him into waiving it.

The third, fourth, and fifth items are both guarantees and procedural reminders. First of all, *you must offer to answer any questions the subject may have and provide instructions as to how to contact someone should questions or problems arise later* [46.116(a)(7)]. As we discussed earlier, this is normally done after the reading of the consent document. But, in addition, you need to put something in the consent form (remember, your subject gets a copy of this) that tells him where to call and who to ask for if he comes up with a question at a later date. Something like this will do: "If you have any further questions after today, please feel free to call 555-3801 and ask for Dr. Smyth."

Second, *you may not have any exculpatory language in the form* [46.116]. In other words, you cannot have any language that waives or appears to waive any of the subject's legal rights, or that releases your institution (or you) from liability for negligence. You may be asking how this squares with the requirement we discussed in the middle section, that the availability (or lack thereof) of compensation and treatment must be stated if the study has a possibility of physical or psychological risk. What happens if compensation or treatment is not available? If you tell the subject this, isn't this using exculpatory language? No, it is not. The presence or absence of compensation or free treatment is information the subject needs to know in order to properly assess the risk. This is quite different from making it seem like the subject is waiving his legal rights or making it seem like the institution is being released from liability for negligence. Phrases like: "The institution assumes no liability for . . . " or "The subject agrees to participate in this experiment at his or her own risk" should never be found in a consent form.

Finally, *you must have a place for the date, a place for the subject to sign, and a place for the witness to sign* [46.117]. Usually, this last item is prefaced by something like: "I, (Printed name), affirm that I have read and understand the above statement and have had all my questions answered."

Now, let's combine our examples and look at a hypothetical ending.

> All information will remain strictly confidential. Although the descriptions and findings of the study may be published, at no time will your name be used. You are at liberty to withdraw your consent at any time without prejudice. If you have any questions after today, please feel free to call 555-3801 and ask for Dr. Smyth.
> --
> I, _____, affirm that I have read and understand the above statement and have had all my questions answered.
>
> Date: _____
>
> Signature: _____
>
> Witness: _____

There it is! That's all there is to it. Just for review, let's combine all our examples from this whole chapter and look at a hypothetical consent form in its entirety on the next page.

CONSENT FORM

The Institute for Counseling Services is carrying out research into various ways of controlling anxiety. We are attempting to determine whether a new biofeedback procedure will work in relieving test anxiety in college freshmen. While we know this procedure is effective with underachieving high school students, it has never been tried on college age students. Your role in this project will consist of attending six one-hour experimental sessions spaced approximately one week apart. Eventually these data will be used to improve the counseling program at West Overshoe Tech.

At these experimental sessions, you will be introduced to a biofeedback relaxation procedure by a staff member who is experienced in this technique. The session itself consists of learning to relax by using a device that tells you how tense or relaxed your muscles are. When this device is connected, it will make clicking sounds. Your job is to sit back, relax, and by relaxing try to make the clicking sounds decrease in frequency. There are no known risks or discomforts associated with this procedure. We have reason to believe that this method may be of significant value in treating test anxiety. However, should you decide not to participate in this project, you will still be eligible for all the regular counseling services.

All information will remain strictly confidential. Although the descriptions and findings may be published, at no time will your name be used. You are at liberty to withdraw your consent to the experiment and discontinue participation at any time without prejudice. If you have any questions after today, please feel free to call 555-3801 and ask for Dr. Smyth.

I, _____, affirm that I have read and understand the above statement and have had all my questions answered.

Date: _____

Signature: _____

Witness: _____

Again, let's try some examples. **Turn to page 97.**

Situation 15

If nothing else, Oddisee is persistent. The beginning and middle sections of his form are fine. He shows you his final paragraph. It reads:

> All information will be kept strictly confidential. Although the descriptions and findings of the study may be published, at no time will your name be used. You are at liberty to withdraw your consent to the experiment and discontinue participation at any time without prejudice. Owing to the nature of this work, we would prefer that you not withdraw once data collection has begun; however, you do have a perfect right to do so. If you have any questions after today, please feel free to contact Mr. Oddisee Wentworth at KL5-8678.
> --
> I, _____, affirm that I have read and understand the above statement and have had all my questions answered.
>
> Date: _____
>
> Signature: _____
>
> Witness: _____

Well, did he get it right this time?

Yes. Turn to page 99.

No. Turn to page 100.

You said, "Yes, Oddisee has finally got it right."
WRONG!

Remember, just a few paragraphs ago we said that the subject has an "inalienable and absolute" right to back out of an experiment at any time? We also said there were no circumstances under which we could pressure him into waiving that right. Oddisee's statement: "Owing to the nature of this work, we would prefer that you not withdraw once data collection has begun . . . " constitutes pressure. You can't do that. You can think it. You can hope it. But you can't say it, infer it, hint at it, and you certainly can't write it in your consent form.

Reread the paragraph stating, "The subject is at liberty to withdraw his or her consent . . . "

Go on to page 101.

You said, "No, Oddisee does not have it right yet."
You are CORRECT.

You interpreted Oddisee's statement, "Owing to the nature of this work we would prefer that you not withdraw once data collection has begun . . . " as constituting pressure on the subject. You also appear to know that this is an absolute no-no.

Very good.

Continue to page 101.

Situation 16

As a young nursing researcher, you have already established yourself as being quite knowledgeable about research ethics. You get a letter from the West Overshoe Medical School. They are testing the behavioral effects of a new tranquilizer and would like you to look over their consent form. You get to the last paragraph and find it reads as follows:

> All data relative to this experiment will be held in strictest confidence. While the findings will be published, at no time will your name or photograph be used without your express permission. In addition, you are free to withdraw your consent and discontinue participation in this project at any time.
> --
> I hereby affirm that I have read and understand the above, that I have had all my questions answered and that I am entering this agreement at my own risk. I will not, therefore, hold the West Overshoe Medical School or its agents liable for any ill effects that may result from my participation in this experiment.
>
> Date: _____ Signature: _____
>
> Printed Name: _____
>
> Witness: _____

Do you tell the medical school that this is all right?

Yes. Turn to page 103.

No. Turn to page 104.

You said, "Yes, I'd tell them it was okay."
WRONG!

The last paragraph was absolutely laced with language relieving the Medical School of any liability and placing all risk on the subject: "... entering this agreement ... at my own risk," "... not hold the West Overshoe Medical School liable ..." etc.

Remember, you can't use any language that waives or appears to waive the subject's legal rights, or which releases the institution or the experimenters from liability for negligence.

Go on to page 105.

You said you would *not* tell the medical school their form was okay.
Very good--you are CORRECT.

The use of exculpatory language in the last paragraph must have been pretty obvious to you, huh? I am glad you remembered that this kind of language cannot be used.

Go on to page 105.

Situation 17

The department chairperson has come back to you with her revised consent form. She shows it to you and again wants your opinion. The last section reads as follows:

> The information you give us will be kept in strict confidence. At no time will your name be used. You are free to terminate your role in the survey and withdraw your consent at any time without prejudice. If you have any questions, please feel free to call Dr. W. B. Grant at 555-5805.
> --
> I, _____, have read and understand the contents of this statement. All of my questions have been answered as of this time. I understand that my participation is voluntary and that I may withdraw at any time.
>
> Signature: _____

Well, did she get it right this time?

Yes. Turn to page 107.

No. Turn to page 108.

You said, "Yes, she has it right this time."
NOPE!
You didn't look close enough. She didn't provide any space for the date and for the witness to sign. This may seem like a trivial thing, but it isn't. It could become very important later on if the experiment (or the experimenter) is ethically or legally challenged and a "who said what to whom" question arises.

Try your hand again. **Turn to page 109.**

You said, "No, she still didn't get it right."
That's RIGHT, she didn't.

Glad to see you didn't fall asleep and fail to notice that there is no place for the date and the signature of the witness. As you know, this information could become very important later on if a question is raised about the ethical or legal propriety of the project.

Good! Try your hand again. **Turn to page 109.**

Situation 18

The conversation you were having with your nursing graduate student on her consent form somehow got off the topic. The cafeteria is now starting to get crowded and you've got a class coming up. So, you get back on track and take a look at the last part of her consent form. It reads:

> All information gathered by this project will be held in strictest confidence. At no point will your name be used on either the curriculum pre- or post-test or on the examination. If at any time you should choose not to continue participation in this project, you are free to withdraw. Should you have any questions with regard to this project or this consent, please feel free to call the university at 555-8366 and ask for Carolyn McArthur.
> --
> I, _____, hereby consent to participate in the project described above. I have read and understand this statement and I have had all my questions answered.
>
> Date: _____ Signature: _____
>
> Witness: _____

You are in a hurry but not so much of a hurry that you can't say:

> *This is excellent. Go ahead and submit it to the Human Subjects Committee--I am sure you'll have no trouble. Turn to page 111.*
>
> *Oops. We've got a problem here. Turn to page 113.*

You said that her form is all right?
You are absolutely RIGHT!

She included all the necessary elements: a statement of confidentiality, permission to withdraw at any time, and an offer to answer any questions. Further, there was no exculpatory language, and she provided a place for the subject's signature, the witness' signature, and the date. Very good. Let's try another.

Turn to page 115.

You said, "Nope, you've got a problem here."

She does? Where?

She included all the necessary elements: a statement of confidentiality, permission to withdraw at any time, and an offer to answer any questions. Further, there was no exculpatory language, and she provided a place for a subject signature, witness signature, and date.

If this section is still causing you problems, reread the chapter opening.

If you think it was just a "temporary lapse," **go on to page 115.**

Situation 19

The more you get into graduate work, the more interesting the field of clinical research seems. For this reason, you were delighted when, in visiting the state mental hospital at West Overshoe, they allowed you to peruse the files of their Institutional Review Board. The project descriptions were fascinating.

Included also in these files, however, were copies of the consent forms used by each of these research projects. Your newly found expertise in research ethics wouldn't let you pass *these* by. One of them had a final section that read:

> If at any time you wish to terminate your participation in this project, you may do so. It is completely voluntary and by withdrawing, you will lose none of your other rights and privileges at this hospital. If you have any questions, please call 555-8366 and ask for Dr. Raymond C. Durban.
>
> Date: _____ Signature: _____
>
> Printed Name: _____
>
> Witness: _____

Is this end section all right?

Yes. Turn to page 117.

No. Turn to page 118.

You said, "Yes, it is all right."

Sorry, it is *not* all right.

Come on, you should have picked up on the fact that the form has no statement concerning the confidentiality of the data.

On the other hand, perhaps you were thrown by the fact that the ending was slightly different. This ending, by the way, is perfectly acceptable. Not every ending has to have, "I, _____, hereby consent to participate . . . " As long as there is a place for the date, the signature of the subject, and the signature of the witness--everything is fine. I would recommend, however, that a place for the subject's printed name appear somewhere. Sometimes signatures can become very illegible.

Turn to page 119.

You said, "No, it is not all right."
CONGRATULATIONS!

I am glad to see you picked up on the fact that there was no statement concerning the confidentiality of the data.

I am also glad to see the change in the ending did not fool you either. Not every form has to end with, "I, _____, hereby consent to participate..." As long as there is a place for the date, the signature of the subject, and the signature of the witness, everything is fine. I would recommend, however, that a place for the subject's printed name appear somewhere. Sometimes signatures can become very illegible.

Turn to page 119.

The Ending   119

Situation 20

One of your students has asked you to chair his dissertation committee. His proposal has been approved, he's made arrangements for subjects, and he has set forth to write the consent form. This is what he finally came up with:

> As part of a dissertation effort in the Department of Psychology at West Overshoe Tech, a study is being conducted on light sensitivity in humans. It involves testing people to find out at what level they first begin to see lights of various colors. This experiment will be conducted in a single half-hour session, and the information may well prove useful in the design of automobile and aircraft warning gauges. While many experiments like this have been done before, this one will involve the use of a new color combination developed here at West Overshoe Tech.
>
> The experiment will involve your sitting in a darkened room and signaling, by pushing a button, the moment you first see a light appear on a panel in front of you. There are no known hazards, risks, or inconveniences associated with this procedure. While there may be no direct benefit to you at this time for participating in this project, we are hopeful that it may eventually lead to the saving of thousands of lives through the improvement of safety instrument lighting.
>
> All information collected will be held in strictest confidence. While this information may be published, at no time will your name be used. In addition, you are free to terminate this consent at any time and withdraw from the project without prejudice. If you have any questions concerning this project or this consent, please feel free to call Kathleen Smyth at 555-5805.
>
> --
>
> I, _____, hereby consent to participate in the project described above. I have read and understand this statement and I have had all my questions answered.
>
> Date: _____   Signature: _____
>
> Witness: _____

Well, how did he do? Is it all right?

Yes. Turn to page 121.

No. Turn to page 122.

You said, "Yes, it's fine."
You are RIGHT again.
The form does indeed contain all the necessary items for a proper consent. May all your future consent forms be as correct as this one.

Turn to page 123.

You said, "No, there is something wrong with it."

NO, the form is just fine. Of course, there may be room for improvement as there is in anything, but the form does meet all the requirements. (Oh well, this is probably the first wrong answer you've given anyway.)

Turn to page 123.

Chapter 6

Consent Form Content: Additional Elements

Occasionally, you will find yourself in a situation where more than minimal risk is involved in a research project and where the subject *must* be given additional information such as the following:

1. The procedure may involve unforeseeable risks.
2. Any significant new findings affecting risk will be reported to the subject.
3. The circumstances for termination of a subject's participation *by the investigator*.
4. Any possible additional costs to the subject.
5. The consequences of a subject's withdrawal from participation.
6. The approximate number of subjects in the study.

In Chapter 4 we talked about letting the subject know what risks he or she might face in the course of the study, what compensation was available, what treatment was available, and so forth. When we went through the examples, however, we spoke about risk factors as if we really *knew* what the risks would be. Well, sometimes we do. On the other hand, sometimes we don't. When we don't, or are not completely sure, we have to inform the subject *that the procedure may involve unforeseen risks* [46.116(b)(1)], using wording such as this: "While we believe there are no substantial risks associated with this study, we cannot say for sure. Because this is such a new area, the possibility of unforeseen risks may exist."

A variation of this circumstance may occur when new findings might change the subject's willingness to participate. If this is a possibility then, again, let the subject know in the consent form. Tell them *that any significant new findings affecting risk will be reported to them*, especially when it comes to therapeutically related research [46.116(b)(5)].

Essentially, these first two items go hand in hand. If there is a possibility of an unknown risk factor, it is also incumbent upon you to inform the subject when those factors become known.

You may recall also that in Chapter 4 we talked about telling the subjects if there were any conditions for participation and in Chapter 5 telling them that they are at liberty to withdraw from the project at any time. Well, these things are still true, but there is another possible circumstance. You might want to be in a position to terminate *their* participation in the study. If you do, you must let them know this in advance--particularly if some monetary reward or other benefit is involved. In other words, you must state *the circumstances for termination of a subject's participation by the investigator* [46.116(b)(2)]. You could say, for example: "Should your scores on the preliminary tests not place you in the desired category, you will be dropped from the study at that point and no payment will be made."

Do you foresee *any possible additional costs to the subject*? If so, let them know what they are likely to be [46.116(b)(3)].

If the subject does elect to drop out of the study, he or she must be informed of *the consequences of a subject's withdrawal from participation* [46.116(b)(4)]. If there are no consequences, that's fine. There is no need to say anything. If there are consequences, however, let them know: "You are free to withdraw your consent to participate in this study at any time. However, if you decide to drop out once treatment has begun, you may experience a period of dizziness and nausea from the sudden withdrawal of the substance we are testing."

Finally, some people might well want to know *the approximate number of subjects in the study* [46.116(b)(6)]. This would be particularly true if you are dealing with especially large or especially small numbers of subjects, and there is more than minimal risk involved.

Keep in mind that the items in this section basically operate off of an ancient, honorable, and occasionally ignored philosophical concept called common sense. You may not run into a study very often that would involve untoward consequences to the subject if he or she were to drop out, but if you did, and *you* were the subject, wouldn't you want to know about them? "Certainly!" I hear you cry.

To be sure you have the concepts down, let's try some examples.

Turn to page 125.

Situation 21

The West Overshoe School of Medicine is working with a new procedure for treating depression called Neurotone. Neurotone consists of passing a low voltage current through the brain. It is a completely painless procedure.

It was devised in the Soviet Union where they report great success with it, but provide very little in the way of side effect or safety information. There could well be some unreported risks connected with it.

You would like to try it out on some of your patients at the West Overshoe Mental Health Clinic where you are a staff physician. The experiment will be done in cooperation with two other research institutions that will be running the same experiment at the same time. You are sent a proposed consent form. The middle section of this consent form reads as follows:

> You will be asked to come to the clinic three times a week for 10 weeks. Your treatment will consist of sitting in a darkened room with a small headset over your ears--very much like a set of earphones--for about 20 minutes each time. These earphones will pass a low voltage current through your head. You will feel no unpleasant sensations from this procedure, other than possibly a slight tingling sensation around your ears. There are no known hazards, inconveniences, or risks involved with this technique. However, you should know that this is a very new procedure to the West, and there may be some hazards or risks we are not aware of at this time. In addition, should some injury occur, you should know that we would not be in a position to offer you any compensation or free treatment. On the other hand, in the Soviet Union this procedure has proven very effective in treating cases of depression similar to yours. Should you decide not to participate in this experiment, however, all the regular treatment and counseling services of the clinic will still be available to you.

So, is this adequate or not?

Yes. Turn to page 127.
No. Turn to page 128.

You said, "Yes, it is adequate."
NOPE!

Remember we said that the procedure might carry with it some unexpected risk. The author of the consent form included that very nicely. But remember that the experiment was being done by two other institutions as well.

Now, let's say that one of these institutions found an unexpected hazard or side effect. That institution would immediately notify the other two (that's simply the way it's done), who would do what? Notify the subjects? Right! But the subjects need to know that. That's something that could very well affect whether or not they might want to participate at all.

Remember, I said a few pages back that unexpected risk and notification of new findings normally go together.

If you are still confused about this, reread the chapter opening.

If you think you've got it straight, **go on to page 129**.

You said, "No, it is not adequate."
You are CORRECT!
You noticed that because the experiment is operating in unclear waters with regard to risk, you need to tell the subjects that there may be unknown hazards *and* that they will be notified should anything turn up.

Very good!

Turn to page 129.

Situation 22

One of the most neglected areas of education is the programming received by the very intelligent child. Most traditional classes are geared for the average student. Most special classes are geared for the below average or handicapped student. The very bright student, however, is usually expected to do well without any special attention.

The Greater Overshoe Consolidated School District has decided to do something about that. A student of yours has been called in as a consultant to design and execute a special program for their very intelligent students. While a formal consent form was not deemed necessary, she knew enough to at least do a "consent letter" to the parents explaining the program and containing all the pertinent elements of a consent form. She did a first draft of the letter and she shows it to you. As you read along you come to the following passage:

> Each student will then be given an intelligence test (the Raven Progressive Matrices test, 3rd edition). Those who score in the top 5% according to the norms of this test will be continued in the experimental program. Those who do not will be dropped from the experimental program and will continue on in their regular classes.

On the one hand, your student does not wish to needlessly make any parents angry. She also doesn't want to have a flawed consent letter either. So, she comes to you. (You see, she knows you had this textbook in graduate school.) She asks whether or not this passage is really necessary. You turn to her with an air of sophisticated, scholarly confidence and say:

"Yes, indeed, my dear. It certainly is." Turn to page 131.

"Tut! Tut! Nothing to worry about." Turn to page 133.

You said, "Yes, indeed, my dear. It certainly is."
You are certainly CORRECT!

You remembered that if there are circumstances in which you might want to terminate a subject's participation in a project--especially if there are benefits to the subject--you need to inform him or her in the consent form (or in this case "consent letter").

Very good.

Turn to page 135.

You said, "Tut! Tut! Nothing to worry about."
WRONG. (Did you really say Tut! Tut!?)
Remember, we said that if you are in a circumstance where you might want to terminate a subject's participation in a project--especially if there are benefits in it for the subject--you need to inform him or her of this fact.

The situation presented here would be a good example. In order to receive the benefits of participating in this experimental program, the students must meet certain criteria. If they don't meet these criteria, there will be no experimental classroom, no benefits. They need to understand this clearly.

If you are still drawing a blank in this area, reread the chapter opening.

When you're finished, **turn to page 135.**

Situation 23

One of your nursing school colleagues has received a small grant to do a series of surveys on the effectiveness of health care delivery systems with unemployed inner-city gang members. In the grant was a provision to pay $10.00 to each subject who underwent two brief interviews spaced one month apart. The money was to be paid only upon completion of the second interview.

He remembered the sage advice you once gave him to keep the design nice and simple. No problem there. You turn to his consent agreement and read the following final paragraph:

> You will be paid $10.00 for helping in this study, and any information you give us will be kept a secret. Your name will not be used on these forms, and no one will ever know what you said. If at any time you want to quit these interviews, you can. It is your choice and no one will force you to come. If you have any questions about any of this, feel free to call 555-7208 and ask for Dr. Robert Garrett.

You look at this young hopeful and say:

"That's fine. See me when you have your data collected." Turn to page 137.

"Son, you're gonna get yourself killed." Turn to page 138.

You said, "That's fine. See me when you have your data collected."
You may never see him again--with or without the data!

Remember the study he's doing? He's going to pay unemployed inner-city gang members $10.00 to do two interviews, but they get paid only if they *complete* the two interviews.

Where in his consent agreement does he say anything about that? Would you like to be the one to explain this little oversight to those kids after they've completed one interview, dropped out, and now show up for their money?

Not me, brother!

Even when dealing with gentler souls, you must always make clear *the consequences of a subject's withdrawal from participation,* if any such consequences exist.

If you missed it, reread the chapter opening and continue on.
If you just didn't like the guy, **go directly to page 139.**

You said, "Son, you're gonna get yourself killed."
You got that right!

You noted that, while his consent agreement promises to pay $10.00 for "helping in this study," it says nothing about having to participate in *both* interview sessions in order to get paid. Trying to explain this little oversight to a group of street youths who show up for payment could become a bit awkward.

You know that you must always specify *the consequences of a subject's withdrawal from participation,* if there are any consequences.

Good job.

Turn to page 139.

After finishing this chapter, you are a certified, bona fide, official writer of proper consent forms, right? Well, maybe...

Remember back in Chapter 2 when I launched into that long sermon about how you should *always design your consent forms so they can be read by your intended subject population?* You may have also noticed that, by and large, the examples we used in learning this material violated this principle. In fact, most of the consent forms we considered were clearly written at the college level. My choice of this writing level was quite intentional. Up to this point, my primary concern has been to get you to read about and write a proper consent form in whatever language was easiest for you to use (presumably college level). But in so doing, we've neglected the aspect of readability. So, before I can *really* pronounce you a certified, bona fide, official writer of proper consent forms, you need to do a few more things.

First, if you haven't already done so, I would like you to now read Appendix B in the back of this book. It outlines three methods of doing a readability test.

Second, I want you to pick out one of the consent forms we used in this book, (say the one on page 95), and apply those tests to it. Use all three of them if you can. Get used to using them.

Third, when you have finished doing this, let's change the game slightly. Let's assume that your subjects are no longer the internationally esteemed, intellectually astute students of West Overshoe Tech. Generally speaking, unless you are doing a study on a known college-educated subject population, your consent forms should never be written much above a tenth grade level and preferably even lower than that. (Keep in mind that newspapers are generally written at about the seventh or eighth grade reading level. That level was not chosen by accident.) Given that, let's see if you can rewrite the form so it can be read by a ninth grader, and confirm that rewrite with a readability test.

When you are finished (come on, do it--don't be lazy), you might want to compare your work with the form I've included in Appendix C. It's a rewrite of the consent document shown on page 95 and is written for about the seventh or eighth grade level.

Then turn to page 141.

CONGRATULATIONS!

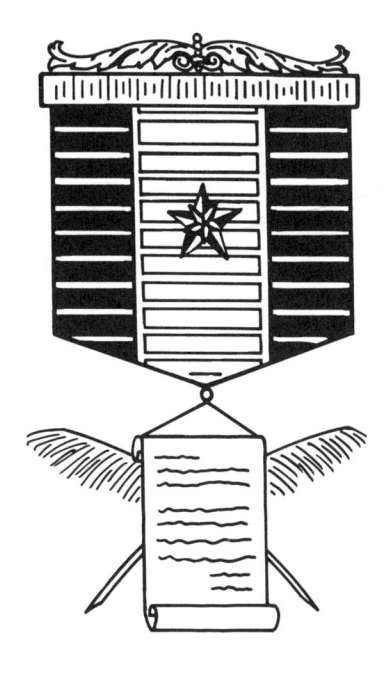

I *now* pronounce you a certified, bona fide, official writer of proper consent forms!

But that's *still* not all there is to it.

Turn to page 143.

Chapter 7

Altering or Waiving Consent

Now that you know how to write and deliver an informed consent, we're going to take a look at how and when *not* to do it. More specifically, we're going to look at those conditions under which you may request that a consent process or its documentation be altered or waived.

Before we examine each guideline separately, however, let's look at them all together.

A consent *procedure* may be altered or waived *by the IRB* if:

1. The research involves no greater than minimal risk.
2. The waiver or alteration will not adversely affect the rights and welfare of the subject.
3. The research could not practically be carried out without the waiver or alteration; and,
4. The subjects will be provided with additional pertinent information after participation.

The *documentation* of the consent process may be waived *by the IRB* if:

1. The consent form is the only record linking the subject to the research and it could potentially be harmful to the subject if the confidentiality of the research were breached; or,
2. The research does not involve more than minimal risk and involves no procedures for which written consent is normally required outside of the research context.

As you can see, these guidelines fall into two natural divisions. In the first group, guidelines 1, 2, 3, and 4 provide the criteria for a consent *process* waiver or alteration, i.e., a change in the way the consent is delivered. The second group deals with conditions under which the IRB can waive or alter the *documentation* of the consent, i.e., a change in the consent form or other written aspect of the consent process.

Altering or Waiving the Consent Process

The first group of guidelines deals with the altering or waiving, by the IRB, of certain aspects of the consent process. Let me repeat a part of that last statement because it's a very important point for you to understand. " . . . altering or waiving, *by the IRB,* of certain aspects of the consent process."

Get it? *You* cannot alter or waive anything! Everything we cover in this chapter is an option *the IRB* has for which you can apply. It is not self-decreed. You have to make a case to the IRB that your humble request for alteration for waiver of the consent form or process is justified. What this chapter is focusing on, then, are the circumstances under which your request *might* be granted (or possibly even ordered) by the IRB.

Perhaps the most important thing that needs to be known about any of these elements is their purpose. These items are not intended to be guidelines for the avoidance of an informed consent. Their intention is just the opposite. They allow the IRB the flexibility to tailor your consent process to the realities of doing research. Take the first set of waiver possibilities, for example.

You know, by now, that to do research with human subjects requires the consent of those subjects, and that the consent must be an informed one. To be an informed one, however, the subject needs to know all about your project. But we also said that there could well be times when, if the subject knew all about your experiment, it would be ruined. There might well be times when your work would require subjects who were naive to the real reasons for your asking them all those questions or whatever you are doing. It is this section of 45 CFR 46 that allows the IRB to waive or alter the normal requirement for full and complete disclosure so that your project can proceed.

The first requirement for this to happen is that your research *must not involve more than minimal risk* [46.116(d)(1)]. As you may recall from the introduction to this book, "minimal risk" refers to research in which the risk of harm is no greater than that found during the course of a normal day or during the course of a routine physical or psychological examination.

Second, the alteration or waiver *will not adversely affect the rights and welfare of the subjects* [46.116(d)(2)]. In some ways, this is a variation of the first requirement, only here we are not talking so much about physical or psychological harm; it refers more to a social harm, if you will. It simply says you can use deception, or whatever you plan to do, but that your subjects may still have certain rights and entitlements. You may not, in any way, adversely affect these or any other aspect of your subject's welfare.

Third, your research has to be such that *the only way you can do the project is by altering or waiving the consent process* [46.116(d)(3)]. If you can find another way of getting the same data that will allow you to proceed with a fully informed consent, then do it that way. Think hard about these alternatives, however, because I assure you, your IRB will. Waivers or alterations are not given lightly.

Finally, if there is any possible way, *provide your subjects with the pertinent information after participation* [46.116(d)(4)]. In other words, if at all possible, hold a "debriefing" with your subjects after the experiment is over. Explain the things you didn't tell them prior to the session and why you had to withhold that information. While the regulations don't require it, I would ask them if it is still all right for you to use the data--sort of a post hoc consent.

In any event, *do whatever is necessary to have them leave feeling good about having participated.* Don't let them leave your presence feeling like they have been lied to, or cheated, or in any other way "had." You not only will lose them as future subjects, you might well lose their data, and you will almost certainly have taken a major step toward giving all researchers a bad name. None of us needs that.

Finally, you should note that 45 CFR 46 contains a series of special provisions for waiving consent procedures if you are doing work on programs that fall under the Social Security Act or other public benefit program [46.116(c)(1) and (2)].

Waiving Consent Documentation

The second group of guidelines deals with the conditions under which the IRB can grant an alteration or a waiver of the *written elements* of the informed consent. It doesn't do away with the consent process; it deals only with the documentation of that process. A waiver or alteration in this area is normally granted for one reason--and one reason only--because it is in the *subject's* best interest to do so. And, even then, unless you are dealing with a special population (see Chapter 8), there are only two circumstances in which it is allowed.

First, a consent documentation waiver is given only if *the consent documentation is the only thing linking the subject and the research and it could be potentially harmful to the subject if the confidentiality of the research were breached* [46.117(c)(1)]. You may recall in Chapter 5 we briefly discussed the problem of confidentiality and how to keep the subject's name from being identified with specific responses. This clause deals with how to keep the subject from being identified with the project *at all*--particularly where that identification could lead to harmful consequences.

The key word here, of course, is *harmful*. Data that could merely be embarrassing is not included in these provisions. For example, research data that could possibly link your subjects to some form of illegal activity would be harmful; data on somebody's snoring habits would not. You might want to use the following as a guideline: If the subjects' participation in your project could place them at risk of criminal or civil liability or be damaging to their financial standing or employability, then you should consider applying for a documentation waiver. Remember from our discussion in Chapter 5, there is almost no way to absolutely guarantee the confidentiality of your data--and that includes your written consent form.

Finally, should you receive a waiver, you are still not free of consent responsibility because (1) you must still go through a verbal consent process with the subjects just as before, and (2) you must then *ask each subject if he or she wants anything in writing that would link him or her to the research.* The subject's decision is final [46.117(c)(1)].

The second circumstance in which a documentation waiver may be given is where you are dealing with *no more than minimal risk,* and you are dealing with research *involving no procedures for which written consent is normally required outside the research context* [46.117(c)(2)]. For example, let's say you are doing a project that involves an experimental approach to a clinical problem but the clinical problem is something that normally *would require* a consent to enable you to deal with it--perhaps a treatment of some kind. What this clause is saying is that, in this situation, the IRB does not have the power to waive the clinical part of the consent, and thus will probably not be able to grant your request.

The last guideline is an important procedural reminder. Even if the written consent is waived, the IRB may still require you to *provide the subjects with a written consent document for their own reference* [46.117(c)(2)]. You see, even with a documentation waiver, the consent *process* must still be carried out. You must prepare the consent form. You must still do the oral presentation. You must still explain to the subjects the option of signing or not signing. And, you must still give them a copy of the form, whether it's signed or not. The only thing that's missing are the names and signatures and, even then, you should offer the subject the opportunity to sign.

Okay? Let's try some examples.

Turn to page 147.

Situation 24

You are on the IRB at the Rehabilitation Center for Alcoholics just outside of West Overshoe. A friend of yours is on staff there and has called to ask your opinion on a research project he is planning.

The project involves testing a new nonaddictive antabuse-like substance that will keep alcoholics from drinking. It works by altering the chemistry of the kidney so that, if the patient ingests alcohol, it will make him or her temporarily violently ill. The only major drawback to it is that, in theory, it could also shut down the kidneys of some people who are susceptible to certain kinds of renal disease.

The subjects consist primarily of chronic alcoholics, many of whom have impaired mental capacities due to their years of drinking. Because of this decreased mental capacity, they want to modify the consent procedure.

Your friend wants to know if that would be possible in this case.

Is it?

Yes, it is possible. Turn to page 149.

No, it is not *possible. Turn to page 150.*

You said, "Yes, it is possible."
You are WRONG.

Remember, one of the rules surrounding the use of these alteration or waiver guidelines is that they can only be used in research carrying no more than minimal risk. Minimal risk is, you'll recall, defined as risk no greater than that found during the course of a normal day or during a routine physical or psychological exam. The substance they plan to test carries the risk of possible kidney shutdown (hardly an everyday occurrence). Therefore, they cannot use an altered consent procedure.

They will probably also have to use the provisions set up for mentally infirm populations, but we haven't gotten to that yet. (See Chapter 8).

Reread the chapter opening, then **go on to page 151.**

You said, "No, it is not possible."

You are CORRECT.

You remembered that one of the rules surrounding the use of these alteration or waiver guidelines was that the project could not involve more than minimal risk. This project, with the possibility of kidney shutdowns occurring in the subjects, is not a minimal risk situation.

Your friend will probably also have to use the guidelines for working with mentally infirm populations (See Chapter 8).

Very good.

Now turn to page 151.

Situation 25

You've just finished advising your friend about the alcoholism study when you get another call. One of the family physicians at the medical school (you have a common IRB arrangement with them) has come to you in a state of alarm.

She was planning to conduct a survey to examine the relationship between heart disease and its impact on the families in a small, dying, New England fishing village. To do this, she was planning to personally interview a large sample of the approximately 1,000 residents. She had obtained a small foundation grant to cover her salary but not enough funds for any additional help. She had organized the data collection procedures, including how she will protect the confidentiality of the data. Suddenly a nasty thought struck her. Even though there were only a thousand people or so in this fishing village, how was she going to get a formal consent from all of them? It would take forever.

She is due to leave in less than two weeks and she appeals to you. Do you think the IRB would allow her to modify the consent procedures to a brief oral statement before each interview?

What do you tell her?

"You can apply for a procedural alteration to the IRB. I am pretty sure you'll get it." Turn to page 153.

"You've got a big problem. It looks like you can't do this study in the amount of time available." Turn to page 155.

You told her, "You can apply for a procedural alteration to the IRB. I am pretty sure you'll get it."

You are RIGHT, she probably will.

She is doing a study which involves no more than minimal risk, it would not adversely affect the subjects at all, and it is a situation where getting a formal consent from all the subjects would make the study practically impossible. Furthermore, there are no procedures involved that would require a consent outside of the research context. I mean, people do surveys all the time.

As long as she does a brief oral consent, I see no reason why the alteration shouldn't be granted.

Nice work. **Turn to page 157.**

You said, "You've got a big problem. It looks like you can't do this study in the amount of time available."

I think you are WRONG.

Why shouldn't she be able to do it? Her study does not involve more than minimal risk, it will not adversely affect her population, and she is quite correct that getting a formal informed consent from all those people *would* make the study almost impossible. Furthermore, there are no procedures involved that would normally require a consent outside the research context. People do surveys all the time.

Remember, the intent of these regulations (all of them) is not to hinder legitimate research or to harass researchers. Their only purpose is to protect human subjects. As long as she is protective of the confidentiality of her data, and does a brief oral consent, I don't think there will be any problem.

Reread the chapter opening, then **turn to page 157.**

Situation 26

Because of your perseverance, foresight, and general good taste in working through this text, you have been asked not only to sit on the West Overshoe Tech IRB, but to serve as witness at a particularly touchy informed consent session.

One of the professors in the WOT School of Social Work is doing a field study of drug pushers (Yes friends, it happens even in West Overshoe!). He plans to use his community connections to interview them on their lifestyle, how they got into the drug selling business, and how they operate.

Obviously, this information will be kept strictly confidential. Indeed, the names of the subjects will not appear on any document, except the consent form. Because of this later requirement, however, he has asked for and received permission to waive the written aspect of the consent.

You are there as he meets his first subject. He gives the person a consent form and goes through the normal consent explanation. As he reaches the end he tells the subject he shouldn't sign the form and explains the reasons why. He asks for questions, receives none, collects the consent form, and begins the interview. You discreetly signal him to meet you in the hall as you quietly slip away.

He puts the interview on hold for a minute, comes out into the hall, and asks you how things went.

What do you say?

"You did just fine." Turn to page 159.

"You did okay, but you made one error." Turn to page 161.

"You did okay, but you made two errors." Turn to page 162.

You said, "You did just fine." You are WRONG.

He missed two very important points in the execution of a waived documentation consent. First, he didn't ask the subject if he *wanted* to waive the signing of the consent form; he told him not to sign it. It's very likely the subject would have passed, but still, he should have asked. It's not hard to envision a case where the subject may *want* a consent form signed by himself and (especially) by a witness.

Second, he did not give the subject a copy of the form. This is important. Even though a signed consent form has not been executed, the subject still has all the same rights. He needs to know those rights and should at least be offered a document to refer to later on.

Reread the section entitled "Waiving Consent Documentation," and **turn to page 163.**

You said, "You did okay, but you made one error."

Close, but no cigar. There were TWO errors. **Turn to page 162** to find out which one you missed.

You said, "You did okay, but you made two errors."

You are right! Very good!

Obviously you noted that he forgot, first of all, to ask the subject if he wanted to sign the consent or not; he simply told him not to sign it. This is important because there could be many circumstances in which the subject would want a consent form that is signed by him and (especially) signed by a witness.

Second, he forgot to give the subject a copy of the consent. Even if the document remains unsigned, the subject still retains all his rights as a subject. He has to know those rights and should at least be offered a consent form to refer to later, should a question arise.

Very good. **Turn to page 163.**

Chapter 8

Working with Special Populations

Working with special populations, such as whom? And why are they special?

Special populations, for purposes of these regulations, are groups such as pregnant women, fetuses, children, prisoners, the elderly, and the mentally infirm. What makes each of these groups "special" is the one thing they hold in common. They all present particular problems in obtaining an informed consent and therefore need at least some comment before we leave this book.

Take pregnant women and fetuses, for example. The woman, assuming she is of adult years and sound mind, can speak for herself. That's no problem. But what about the fetus she is carrying? Does the fetus have rights? 45 CFR 46 says it does and you need to be aware of them.

Do children need to be consulted before you can use them in research activities, or is parental permission enough? 45 CFR 46 says you don't need to get their consent, but you do need to get their *assent*. There is a difference, and we'll explain what that difference is.

Or what about prisoners? How do you get a *freely given* consent from a person who is living in an inherently coercive environment? Is it possible? 45 CFR 46 says it is, but you have to take certain precautions.

Finally, we must discuss the mentally infirm and certain classes of elderly, special populations, indeed. How do you get an informed consent when you are doing research on a population specifically *because* they have decreased or altered mentation? What about the elderly? They must be given an informed consent too. But what do you do if, because of their age, they do not think as clearly as they once did? Strangely, the issue of mentally infirm populations is the one area about which 45 CFR 46 is silent--at least for the time being. That is not, however, the same thing as saying you are ethically off the hook. I will give you some thoughts on precautions you might take in working with these populations.

So, let's take them in order, starting with pregnant women.

Research Involving Pregnant Women

The pregnant woman is an informed consent problem for two reasons. First, because of the nature of her condition, she is at a particularly vulnerable moment in her life where psychological or physical dependence on the medical establishment is very possibly at an all time high. Secondly, there are two people to be considered here--the mother and the fetus--and, at least according to the regulations, the fetus has some rights in the matter. Because of these factors, a number of general provisions have been made that are *in addition to* all the other things that can be found in 45 CFR 46.

The following are some "cannots" to keep in mind. You *cannot* use a pregnant woman in a research project unless:

1. All appropriate studies on animals and nonpregnant women have been completed [46.206(a)(1)].

2. The purpose of the study is to meet the health needs of the mother or the fetus, the risk to the fetus is minimal, and the mother and fetus are placed in the least possible risk situation that is consistent with meeting the objectives of the study [46.206(a)(2) and 46.207(a)].

3. The mother and father are competent and have given their informed consent. The informed consent, however, *must* carry with it full information regarding the possible impact of the procedure on the fetus [46.207(b)].

Now, doubtless you have spotted the phrase "mother *and* father" in the third item above. It means what it says, friends. Mother *and* father. But what if you don't know who the father is, or can't find him? That's covered too.

You can go with a mother-only consent if: (1) the purpose of the activity is to meet the health needs of the mother; (2) the father's identity or whereabouts cannot be reasonably known; (3) he is not reasonably available; or, (4) the pregnancy is the result of rape [46.207(b)]. (It doesn't say anything about incest, though. I imagine that will change in later versions.)

Next, if the study involves terminating the pregnancy, no one involved in the study can be a part of any decisions as to (1) the timing, method, and procedures of the termination; or (2) the viability of the fetus after termination. In addition, you can't use the termination process as part of your research if it causes more than minimal risk to either the mother or the fetus [46.206(a)(3) and (4)].

Finally, you can offer no inducements, monetary or any other kind, to terminate the pregnancy [46.206(b)].

Research Involving Fetuses

The regulations regarding fetuses make a distinction as to whether the fetus is still inside the womb (*in utero*) or outside the womb (*ex utero*).

If the fetus is still inside the womb, the precautions pretty closely parallel those for pregnant women. You cannot do research on an *in utero* fetus unless (1) the purpose of the research is to meet the health needs of the particular fetus, and the fetus will be placed at risk only to the extent necessary to meet those needs; or (2) the risk to the fetus is minimal and the study is designed to obtain important biomedical knowledge that cannot be obtained in any other way. In addition, as above, the mother and father must be legally competent, and you must get their informed consent [46.208(a) and (b)].

If the fetus is *outside* the womb, things get a bit more complicated because you need to determine whether the fetus is viable or not. What constitutes viability, however, is provided for you by the regulations. First of all, a *fetus* is defined as the product of conception from the time of implantation (i.e., when someone gets pregnant) to the point that a determination is made that the fetus is viable [46.203(c)]. A *viable fetus* is a fetus that, after delivery, is able to survive (given available medical therapy) to the point of independently maintaining heartbeat and respiration. A *nonviable* fetus is one that can't maintain these functions [46.203(d) and (e)].

Given these definitions of viability and nonviability, this is the research that can and cannot be done on fetuses. Until you know that the fetus is *viable*, there isn't much you can do in the way of experimentation. The only exception to this is if: (1) what you are going to do involves no added risk to the fetus, and it will develop important biomedical knowledge which can't be obtained any other way; or, (2) the purpose of the experiment is to help the fetus to survive to the point of viability [46.209(a)(1) and (2)]. If the fetus is clearly *not viable*, you can use it for experimentation as long as your experiment doesn't attempt to artificially maintain its vital functions, or the reverse, attempt to artificially terminate its vital functions. Also, the purpose of the experiment has to be to yield important biomedical knowledge that can't be obtained any other way [46.209(b)(1)-(3)]. Whether the fetus is viable or not, you must get an informed consent from both the mother and father, as described earlier [46.209(d)].

Research Involving Children

The next category of special populations has to do with children and is, by far, the most complicated. The reason for this is because there are so many factors to consider. We'll take them one at a time and try to make things as clear as possible.

To begin with, there are those "exempted categories" we talked about briefly in the introduction. Even if your IRB is honoring these exemptions for all other research, children are an exception. Specifically, if you plan to do research involving survey or interview procedures with children, your project will fall under 45 CFR 46. The same is true if you plan to do research involving the observation of public behavior in which you are not a part of the activities being observed. [46.401(b)]. Secondly, what you have to do for an informed consent will vary depending on what the level of risk is and what benefits are likely to accrue to the child. We'll start with the easiest situation.

You may remember back in the introduction we said the regulations defined "minimal risk" as being risks of harm that are no greater, considering probability and magnitude, than those ordinarily encountered in daily life or during the performance of routine physical or psychological examination or tests [46.102(g)]. So if your project involves no greater than minimal risk as defined here, all you need to do is get the permission of *one* parent or guardian and the assent of the child [46.404 and 46.408(b)].

But, wait a minute, what exactly is meant by "permission"? What's meant by "parents or guardian"? What's meant by "assent," and what's the cut-off point for what constitutes a "child"? 45 CFR 46 comes to the rescue.

Most of these terms mean pretty much what you would expect them to mean. A "parent" is a child's biological or adoptive parent [46.402(d)]. A "guardian" is an individual who is authorized under applicable state or local law to consent on behalf of the child to general medical care [46.402(e)]. And "permission" is the agreement of the parent(s) or guardian(s) to allow the child to participate in your research [46.402(c)]. While it doesn't explicitly say so in the regulations, I interpret "permission" to mean an informed consent by the parent or guardian [46.408(b)]. You may also want to note that the IRB can waive the permission requirement completely in order to protect the child (for example, if you were working with abused or neglected children) [46.408(c)].

But then there are those other terms, "assent," and what exactly is a "child" anyway? The federal government labored long and hard over the issue of exactly when a child becomes an adult for purposes of consenting to participate in research. All sorts of ages were suggested, and many ponderous tomes by assorted educational psychologists were submitted. What the government eventually did, however, was to punt on the issue. A child is a person who has " . . . not attained the legal age for consent to treatments or procedures involved in the research, under the applicable law in which the research will be conducted" [46.402(a)]. In other words, go look it up. For most projects, the "applicable law" will be state law, but there may be additional local or alternate state rulings to be considered as well, so we would advise you to check with your IRB for the exact rulings pertaining to your area.

Finally, there is the matter of "assent." The parents must give consent; the child must give assent. All that means is that you must outline to the child, in terms appropriate to that child, what it is you plan to do and why. The child must then agree to be a part of it. But note that this must be an affirmative statement. The kid has to say it's okay. Just because he or she didn't say you couldn't, doesn't mean you can [46.402(b)]. Your IRB will inform you as to how you are supposed to document this assent [46.408(e)].

The IRB is also supposed to determine whether the children involved are capable of providing assent. To determine that, they will be looking at their ages, maturity levels, and psychological state. If they determine that the children cannot reasonably be consulted or that the procedure is of such potential benefit to them, they can rule that the child's assent is *not* a necessary condition for proceeding with the research. But here again, notice that *the IRB must do the waiving*--not you [46.408(a)].

All right, so we've got that straightened out. If your project involves no greater than minimal risk, all you need is the permission of one parent or guardian, the assent of the child, and you're off and running.

But there are times when the risks may exceed minimal. If that occurs, things will change, depending on whether the research presents the prospect of directly benefiting the child or not. If the research presents the prospect of direct benefit to the child, you can do this type of research only if (1) the risk is justified by the potential direct benefit to the subject; (2) the risk-benefit ratio is at least as good as that presented by available alternate approaches; and, again, (3) you have the permission of at least one of the parents and the assent of the child [46.405 and 46.408(b)].

If there is greater than minimal risk, but presenting no prospect of direct benefit to the child, the research will be a bit stickier, but can be done if (1) the risk involved is only a minor increase over minimal risk; (2) the procedures you plan to use are not a horror show--that is, they are reasonably commensurate with those inherent in a medical, dental, psychological, social, or educational situation; (3) the research is likely to yield important generalizable knowledge about the subject's disorder or condition; and (4) you have the permission of *both* of the parents and the assent of the child (notice I said *both* parents) [46.406 and 46.408(b)].

Finally there is the ultimate: research which is not otherwise approvable, but which presents an opportunity to understand, prevent, or alleviate a serious problem affecting the health or welfare of children. If this is what you have in mind, make friends with your IRB because you're going to need all the help you can get. You can get approval for this kind of thing, but it has to come from The Secretary--as in, The Secretary of Health and Human Services--as in, 10 people removed from being President. It works like this.

First, you need to secure agreement from your IRB that your project indeed presents a reasonable opportunity to further the understanding, prevention, or alleviation of a serious problem affecting children. Then it will be sent to Washington, D.C., where the Secretary will convene a panel of experts in areas such as science, medicine, education, ethics, and law to look your proposal over and put it out for public review and comment. After this public review is completed, the responses will be collated and your project will be adjudicated. Nothing to it [46.407].

The final area--lest you should think anything might fall through the cracks--is when you are working with children who are wards of the state or of some other agency. Again, they can be subjects but (1) the work must be related to their status as wards; or (2) it must be done at a school, hospital, camp, or whatever, in which the majority of subjects *are not* wards [46.409(a)(1)-(2)].

If your project meets one of these two conditions, you have to do one other thing. You must obtain an advocate for each ward who is to be a part of the study. They must be someone apart from whomever else may be acting on behalf of the child as a guardian or in loco parentis.

Now don't panic. One individual can serve as advocate for more than one child, but the person has to be someone who has an appropriate background and experience and who agrees to act in the best interests of the child for the duration of your experiment. The person also cannot be connected in any way with your project, you, or the guardian organization [46.409(b)].

Working with Prisoners

The central issue surrounding informed consent and prison populations is this: can a person who is involuntarily confined in a prison or other penal institution ever *freely give* an informed consent? According to the interpretations given to a 1973 court ruling, the answer is no. Does that mean that we cannot do research on prison populations? No, it doesn't mean that at all. But you *do* have to do it the way 45 CFR 46 says.

To begin with, let's define what we mean by a "prisoner." According to the regulations, a prisoner is any individual involuntarily confined in a penal institution. This includes not only people confined in what we normally think of as prisons, but people detained in alternative programs or facilities, and people detained pending arraignment, trial, or sentencing [46.303(c)]. The operative word here is "involuntary." With the exclusion of those confined in mental hospitals (which we'll deal with below), if the subject population is involuntarily detained, they probably qualify as "prisoners" for purposes of these regulations.

Secondly, you will probably have to use more than one IRB--the IRB you would normally go to, plus another with a slightly different composition. This second IRB will most likely be found at the institution in which you want to do your work, and you will find that the majority of its members will have no connection with the prison (other than being on the IRB) and at least one of the members will be a prisoner [46.304].

To do the work, you will have to provide certain guarantees. You will have to be sure, first, that any possible advantages accruing to the prisoner will not be so much, when compared to the general living conditions of the place, that it would affect his or her ability to weigh the risk of the research against those benefits. Second, the risks involved must be commensurate with the kinds of risks that would be acceptable to non-prisoner volunteers. Third, the selection of the prisoners must be fair. Fourth, the informed consent must be presented in a language that is understandable to the subject population (but having read this book, you should have no problem with that). Fifth, and most importantly, you have to make it perfectly clear to the prisoners that their participation in your project will have *no effect* on whether or not they get parole. In fact, the parole board will not even know that they have been participants. Finally, you have to be able to guarantee follow-up care, and the prisoners have to be so informed [46.305(a)(2)-(7)].

Given these assurances, you will now be able to do your work--within limits--because there are only four kinds of research that are permissible [46.306(a)-(d)].

1. Studies of the possible causes, effects, and processes of incarceration and of criminal behavior, provided the study represents no more than minimal risk and minimal inconvenience.

2. Studies of prisons as institutional structures or of prisoners as incarcerated persons, provided the research represents no more than minimal risk and inconvenience.

3. Studies that deal with topics that particularly affect prisoners as a class (e.g., hepatitis studies or studies dealing with alcoholism, drug addiction, sexual assaults, etc.), but only if approved by the Secretary of Health and Human Services.

4. Studies that deal with practices that have the intent and reasonable probability of improving the health or well-being of the subject. And, even here, if you use control groups which may not receive any benefits, the study must be approved by the Secretary.

Research Involving the Mentally Infirm and the Elderly

I know I have some of you disagreeing with me already on this section, and I haven't even said anything yet. In the title I used the term "mentally infirm," and there are those who would argue that this is not an appropriate term--that it is not in current clinical use, that it is pejorative in nature, that it is inaccurate or incomplete, etc. They are probably right on all counts. The problem is that neither I, nor anyone else I know of, has come up with a term that's any better.

This issue also gives you a pretty good indicator of the state of the ethical art with regard to working with these populations. Getting consensus on what steps need to be taken when working with elderly and (better get used to it) mentally infirm populations has proven to be an elusive goal. The procedures that *have* been suggested by various groups and persons have universally found opposition from one quarter or another. This is also one reason why you not only don't find any mention of working with these populations in 45 CFR 46 but, as of this writing, you will not be likely to find anything in the near future. It is a very complex topic. Just think about one small aspect of it. How exactly *do* you go about obtaining a *truly informed consent* from a population that you want to study specifically because their mental processes are askew? It's a contradiction in terms and yet, somehow, it has to be done. Somehow, their rights must be protected.

Having no qualms about tromping around where angels fear to tread, I will endeavor to provide you with at least *some* guidelines you may find useful. They are *not* based on 45 CFR 46 nor on any other body of law. They are simply items I have picked up along the way from various sources and commend to you.

One source upon which I will be relying heavily was mentioned in the historical background in Chapter 1, namely, the National Commission for the Protection of Human Subjects of Biomedical and Behavioral Research. I highly recommend you read their report on "Research Involving Those Institutionalized as Mentally Infirm" and its appendix.

All right. Let's begin with a clarification of the term I used above, "mentally infirm." This is one of those terms where just about everyone knows what you're talking about even if *they* can't precisely define it either. I am referring to people who are psychotic, retarded, senile, brain damaged, or have any other substantial impairment of their mental functioning. Now, a Philadelphia lawyer could probably bring that definition to its knees in about 10 seconds, but there it is. If you are planning to do a research project on individuals who fall into one or more of these categories there are, first, some general cautions I would propose and, second, some specific advice I would offer concerning doing the informed consent.

Some general cautions:

1. Do not use this population unless you absolutely have to--especially if they are institutionalized. Use them *only* if the only way you can meet the objectives of your research is by including them. Using them simply because they are handy is a no-no. That's called exploitation.

2. Use the group with the least degree of disability that is consistent with the objectives of your research. For example, never use a profoundly re-

tarded population if you can accomplish the same objectives by using an educable retarded group, and never use an educable retarded group if you could just as easily use a group of slow learners.

3. If you are going to take biological samples of any kind (e.g., blood or urine samples) or you are going to do testing (e.g., intelligence or psychological tests), always use existing data that has been gathered for other diagnostic or therapeutic purposes, if at all possible.

4. Participation in your project should never interfere with patient care, unless it is absolutely necessary to meet the goals of your study.

5. Privacy and confidentiality are critical. Remember that, for some, the very fact that they are in a study dealing with the mentally infirm could be harmful information if it got out.

6. Make sure your design is tight and your procedures are safe. Remember, a population with diminished mental capacity often has a diminished capacity to object.

7. Do not use your own clinical population as your experimental group unless you absolutely must. The difficulty here is twofold. First, you will be running up against a possible conflict of interest problem in that you will be simultaneously in a protective role (as their therapist or physician) as well as being the person in charge of getting the experiment done. Secondly, it is very difficult for some people to decline to participate in a study if it is *their* therapist or physician who is asking them to participate. They must feel perfectly free to decline if that is what they want to do.

8. USE A WITNESS AT ALL CONSENT PROCEEDINGS. Ideally, this witness should be someone who is a professional working with your population and who has no particular interest in, or connection with, your project. There are a number of reasons for this, which I will list below.

9. Finally, a note from hard experience: if you are doing a project in an institutional setting, don't forget that the point of the patient being in that setting is to eventually get out. Keep that in mind when you are designing a long-term study or you may wind up with an attrition rate that will make your data worthless.

The trickiest part of the whole process, however, is the informed consent. One of the major things that makes it so tricky are the degrees of infirmity you might find--sometimes within the same population--each one calling for a slightly different consent approach.

Two of the hardest populations to work with in this regard are the mentally infirm and the elderly. Within either group you could easily find anything from persons with totally intact mentation, to people whose cognitive functions have completely shut down. Worse (from a consent standpoint), you could easily find some people who function perfectly well in some cognitive areas but not in others, and worse yet, some who function perfectly well in some cognitive areas *on some days* but not on others. (Do you see what we mean by complex?) In view of this and in view of the lack of hard and fast federal guidelines in place, I will offer you only some general guidelines of my own. As we have mentioned many times previously in this book, however, *contact your local IRB for the final word on what you can and cannot do in your specific situation.*

In general, whenever you are doing a consent with a mentally impaired population--*have a witness*. As mentioned above, this witness should be a professional at working with your particular population and should not be connected in any way to your project.

Now, I know we talked about having witnesses to all consent processes earlier in the book. I have also been around enough to know that it is often not done. For this population, however, *do it* because you are going to ask the witness to perform three very important functions.

First, you are going to ask the witness to attest to the fact that a consent occurred at all. At a minimum, you need to be able to demonstrate that.

Second, you should ask the witness to attest to the fact that the individual subject was, in his or her opinion, capable of giving consent at that moment. Remember the problem we mentioned earlier of the extreme variability in cognitive function that you can find in the elderly and mentally infirm? This is a partial answer to that problem. There is no way I know to scientifically and systematically determine whether a person is capable of giving consent or not. There is no quick pencil and paper test. There is no machine to which we can connect them. In the final analysis, whether a person is capable of giving consent is going to be a subjective judgment. Fine. Just don't let that judgment be yours alone. That's where the witness comes in. If there is a conflict where you think the subject is capable and the witness does not, the witness wins.

Third, if the subject is incapable, you may still need to get his or her assent (see below) as opposed to consent. If that is the case, your witness will need to attest that the assent was given.

Okay, so now you have your witness in place. Now what? How do you go about getting the consent? Let's take several situations in order from the least difficult to most difficult. Let's start with studies that involve the subject in *no greater than minimal risk.*

Subject is capable of giving consent. If, in the opinion of yourself and your witness, the subject's ability to understand and judge the elements of the consent process is unimpaired, then there is no problem. Just carry out the consent process just as I have outlined earlier in the book. Please pay particular attention to the readability of your consent form and the complexity of the language you use. While your population may be capable of giving consent, that is not the same thing as saying that there is no decrease at all in mental capabilities. Go easy.

Subject is NOT capable of giving consent, but IS capable of giving assent. I know. Your first question is "where is the cut-off point between being able to give consent and giving assent?" My answer is that I don't know--at least not exactly. If your subjects' capacity to understand and judge is apparently impaired, yet they are still able to otherwise generally function, they probably fall into this category. According to the National Commission, the standard for assent should contain four things: (1) that the subject know what procedures will be performed in the research; (2) that he or she be able to choose freely to undergo those procedures; (3) that he or she be able to communicate those choices unambiguously; and, (4) that he or she be aware that subjects may withdraw from participation. If your subjects can't do at least those things, keep reading.

Subject is NOT capable of assent. If, in the opinion of yourself or your witness, your subject is not capable of giving assent as defined above, then the absence of objection should be sufficient IF (a big IF) there is *no more than minimal risk involved.* If they do object, however, or there is *more than minimal risk*, then you should only proceed if it is *to the subject's benefit to participate* and you get approval from a court of competent jurisdiction.

Not all studies are designed to directly benefit the immediate subject population. Often you find yourself working on solutions to problems that you hope will someday benefit others, but will be of no real value to those who already have the problem. Here is where things get dicey--especially if *more than minimal risk is involved.* Let's again take them one at a time.

More than minimal risk WITH direct benefit. In these circumstances, follow the consent/assent procedures as outlined above. Just be sure that the risk is justified by the expected benefits; in other words, that it is at least as favorable as that presented by alternative approaches.

More than minimal risk with NO direct benefit. Here again, follow the consent/assent steps outlined above but be sure of two things. First, that the knowledge you are going after is justified by the risk you are imposing; and second, if the subject is incapable of assenting and actively objects to participating, drop it. Don't do the study, or at least don't use that subject. (You probably aren't going to get very good data anyway.)

Above all, any time you are working with mentally infirm populations, *work very closely with your IRB.* Let them help you. As we mentioned above, there are no federal regulations to provide guidance for your work. Ethically speaking, you will be flying by the seat of your pants. Don't do it alone.

Chapter 9

A Final Summing-Up

So far we have looked a bit at the regulatory history surrounding human experimentation, and we have looked in some detail at the laws that currently govern it in this country. In the process, we have touched on the basics of the IRB system and how it works. These discussions contributed to our main purpose, learning how to design and deliver an informed consent. Finally, we saw how the consent process must be altered when working with special populations. Throughout the book, however, our information has been derived mostly from 45 CFR 46, the part of the Code of Federal Regulations that governs human experimentation. Therein lies both the strength and the weakness of the book and of the IRB system itself.

In my opinion, 45 CFR 46 is one of the most thoughtful, carefully constructed sets of governmental regulations in existence. It strikes a marvelous balance between the interests of a public that must be afforded certain rights, and a scientific community that must be afforded certain prerogatives. That is its strength.

Its weakness lies in the fact that the delivery mechanism is basically a list of rules. You must do this. You may do that. Thing X can be done under certain circumstances but not under others. How do you design a set of specific rules that will cover all men, at all times, under all circumstances? The answer, of course, is that you cannot. There will always be the project that doesn't quite fit the rules, the project that has a certain twist to it or that delves into an area that was completely unanticipated by the framers of 45 CFR 46. What do you do then?

Part of the answer, at least for the researcher, is to simply ask the IRB for guidance, though in many ways, that begs the question. It is true that one of the primary functions of the IRB is to put the element of human judgment into the system. While that is important, it only raises another question. How is the IRB supposed to know what do do? Your local IRB is not a convention of philosopher-kings. It is composed of researchers, administrators, physicians, lawyers, clergymen, laypersons, and other people just like yourself. The federal government anticipated this problem and the need for a philosophical un-

176 Informed Consent: A Tutorial

derpinning to the regulations--some general principles that could guide both the researchers and the IRBs in all their deliberations, but especially when considering those cases that "don't quite fit."

You may recall from Chapter 1 that, in the mid-1970s, the National Commission for the Protection of Human Subjects of Biomedical and Behavioral Research was formed. The function of this group was to study in depth the issues involved in conducting research with human subjects and to make specific recommendations as to what would be included in the regulations. In order to develop some general principles, the commission went on an intensive four-day retreat to the Smithsonian Institution's Belmont Conference Center. There, they drafted a document that would " . . . provide federal employees, members of Institutional Review Boards and scientific investigators with . . . an analytical framework that will guide the resolution of ethical problems arising from research involving human subjects." The result of these deliberations is known as the Belmont Report and is reproduced below in its entirety.

The report begins by discussing the difference between research and practice. It then goes on to propose three general principles to keep in mind when constructing or reviewing research with human subjects, entitled respect for persons, beneficence, and justice. After describing what is meant by each of these principles, it then illustrates how these principles can be applied to the areas of informed consent, risk/benefit assessment, and the selection of subjects of research.

Although you should know and apply all the rules and regulations outlined earlier in this book, if you come away with nothing but the ability to apply the Belmont principles to your work, you will not go wrong in the ethical conduct of your research no matter what rules, regulations, codes, or covenants are currently in effect.

The Belmont Report: Ethical Principles and Guidelines for Research Involving Human Subjects

Scientific research has produced substantial social benefits. It has also posed some troubling ethical questions. Public attention was drawn to these questions by reported abuses of human subjects in biomedical experiments, especially during the Second World War. During the Nuremberg War Crimes Trials, the Nuremberg Code was drafted as a set of standards for judging physicians and scientists who had conducted biomedical experiments on concentration camp prisoners. This code became the prototype of many later codes* intended to as-

---

* Since 1945, various codes for the proper and responsible conduct of human experimentation in medical research have been adopted by different organizations. The best known of these codes are the Nuremberg Code of 1947, the Helsinki Declaration of 1964 (revised in 1975), and the 1971 Guidelines (codified into Federal Regulations in 1974) issued by the U.S. Department of Health,

sure that research involving human subjects would be carried out in an ethical manner.

The codes consist of rules, some general, others specific, that guide the investigators or the reviewers of research in their work. Such rules often are inadequate to cover complex situations; at times they come into conflict, and they are frequently difficult to interpret or apply. Broader ethical principles will provide a basis on which specific rules may be formulated, criticized and interpreted.

Three principles, or general prescriptive judgments, that are relevant to research involving human subjects are identified in this statement. Other principles may also be relevant. These three are comprehensive, however, and are stated at a level of generalization that should assist scientists, subjects, reviewers and interested citizens to understand the ethical issues inherent in research involving human subjects. These principles cannot always be applied so as to resolve beyond dispute particular ethical problems. The objective is to provide an analytical framework that will guide the resolution of ethical problems arising from research involving human subjects.

This statement consists of a distinction between research and practice, a discussion of the three basic ethical principles, and remarks about the application of these principles.

A. Boundaries Between Practice and Research

It is important to distinguish between biomedical and behavioral research, on the one hand, and the practice of accepted therapy on the other, in order to know what activities ought to undergo review for the protection of human subjects of research. The distinction between research and practice is blurred partly because both often occur together (as in research designed to evaluate a therapy) and partly because notable departures from standard practice are often called "experimental" when the terms "experimental" and "research" are not carefully defined.

For the most part, the term "practice" refers to interventions that are designed solely to enhance the well-being of an individual patient or client and that have a reasonable expectation of success. The purpose of medical or behavioral practice is to provide diagnosis, preventive treatment or therapy to particular individuals.* By contrast, the term "research" designates an activity

---

Education, and Welfare. Codes for the conduct of social and behavioral research have also been adopted, the best known being that of the American Psychological Association, published in 1973.

* Although practice usually involves interventions designed solely to enhance the well-being of a particular individual, interventions are sometimes applied to one individual for the enhancement of the well-being of another (e.g., blood donation, skin grafts, organ transplants) or an intervention may have the dual purpose of enhancing the well-being of a particular individual, and, at the same

designed to test a hypothesis, permit conclusions to be drawn, and thereby to develop or contribute to generalizable knowledge (expressed, for example, in theories, principles, and statements of relationships). Research is usually described in a formal protocol that sets forth an objective and a set of procedures designed to reach that objective.

When a clinician departs in a significant way from standard or accepted practice, the innovation does not, in and of itself, constitute research. The fact that a procedure is "experimental," in the sense of new, untested or different, does not automatically place it in the category of research. Radically new procedures of this description should, however, be made the object of formal research at an early stage in order to determine whether they are safe and effective. Thus, it is the responsibility of medical practice committees, for example, to insist that a major innovation be incorporated into a formal research project.*

Research and practice may be carried on together when research is designed to evaluate the safety and efficacy of a therapy. This need not cause any confusion regarding whether or not the activity requires review; the general rule is that if there is any element of research in an activity, that activity should undergo review for the protection of human subjects.

B. Basic Ethical Principles

The expression "basic ethical principles" refers to those general judgments that serve as a basic justification for the many particular ethical prescriptions and evaluations of human actions. Three basic principles, among those generally accepted in our cultural tradition, are particularly relevant to the ethics of research involving human subject: the principles of respect for persons, beneficence and justice.

1. Respect for Persons

Respect for persons incorporates at least two basic ethical convictions: first, that individuals should be treated as autonomous agents, and second, that per-

---

time, providing some benefit to others (e.g., vaccination, which protects both the person who is vaccinated and society generally). The fact that some forms of practice have elements other than immediate benefit to the individual receiving an intervention, however, should not confuse the general distinction between research and practice. Even when a procedure applied in practice may benefit some other person, it remains an intervention designed to enhance the well-being of a particular individual or groups of individuals; thus, it is practice and need not be reviewed as research.

* Because the problems related to social experimentation may differ substantially from those of biomedical and behavioral research, the Commission specifically declines to make any policy determination regarding such research at this time. Rather, the Commission believes that the problem ought to be addressed by one of its successor bodies.

sons with diminished autonomy are entitled to protection. The principles of respect for persons thus divides into two separate moral requirements: the requirement to acknowledge autonomy and the requirement to protect those with diminished autonomy.

An autonomous person is an individual capable of deliberation about personal goals and of acting under the direction of such deliberation. To respect autonomy is to give weight to autonomous persons' considered opinions and choices while refraining from obstructing their actions unless they are clearly detrimental to others. To show a lack of respect for an autonomous agent is to repudiate that person's considered judgments, to deny an individual the freedom to act on those considered judgments, or to withhold information necessary to make a considered judgment, when there are no compelling reasons to do so.

However, not every human being is capable of self-determination. The capacity for self-determination matures during an individual's life, and some individuals lose this capacity wholly or in part because of illness, mental disability, or circumstances that severely restrict liberty. Respect for the immature and the incapacitated may require protecting them as they mature or while they are incapacitated.

Some persons are in need of extensive protection, even to the point of excluding them from activities which may harm them; other persons require little protection beyond making sure they undertake activities freely and with awareness of possible adverse consequences. The extent of protection afforded should depend upon the risk of harm and the likelihood of benefit. The judgment that any individual lacks autonomy should be periodically reevaluated and will vary in different situations.

In most cases of research involving human subjects, respect for persons demands that subjects enter into the research voluntarily and with adequate information. In some situations, however, application of the principle is not obvious. The involvement of prisoners as subjects of research provides an instructive example. On the one hand, it would seem that the principle of respect for persons requires that prisoners not be deprived of the opportunity to volunteer for research. On the other hand, under prison conditions they may be subtly coerced or unduly influenced to engage in research activities for which they would not otherwise volunteer. Respect for persons would then dictate that prisoners be protected. Whether to allow prisoners to "volunteer" or to "protect" them presents a dilemma. Respecting persons, in most hard cases, is often a matter of balancing competing claims urged by the principle of respect itself.

2. Beneficence

Persons are treated in an ethical manner not only by respecting their decisions and protecting them from harm, but also by making efforts to secure their well-being. Such treatment falls under the principle of beneficence. The term "beneficence" is often understood to cover acts of kindness or charity that go beyond strict obligation. In this document, beneficence is understood in a stronger sense, as an obligation. Two general rules have been formulated as complementary expressions of beneficent actions in this sense: 1) do not harm and 2) maximize possible benefits and minimize possible harms.

The Hippocratic maxim "do not harm" has long been a fundamental principle of medical ethics. Claude Bernard extended it to the realm of research, saying that one should not injure one person regardless of the benefits that might come to others. However, even avoiding harm requires learning what is harmful; and, in the process of obtaining this information, persons may be exposed to risk of harm. Further, the Hippocratic Oath requires physicians to benefit their patients "according to their best judgment." Learning what will in fact benefit may require exposing persons to risk. The problem posed by these imperatives is to decide when it is justifiable to seek certain benefits despite the risks involved, and when the benefits should be foregone because of the risks.

The obligations of beneficence affect both individual investigators and society at large, because they extend both to particular research projects and to the entire enterprise of research. In the case of particular projects, investigators and members of their institutions are obliged to give forethought to the maximization of benefits and the reduction of risk that might occur from the research investigation. In the case of scientific research in general, members of the larger society are obliged to recognize the longer term benefits and risks that may result from the improvement of knowledge and from the development of novel medical, psychotherapeutic, and social procedures.

The principle of beneficence often occupies a well-defined justifying role in many areas of research involving human subjects. An example is found in research involving children. Effective ways of treating childhood diseases and fostering healthy development are benefits that serve to justify research involving children--even when individual research subjects are not the direct beneficiaries. Research also makes it possible to avoid the harm that may result from the application of previously accepted routine practices that on closer investigation turn out to be dangerous. But the role of the principle of beneficence is not always so unambiguous. A difficult ethical problem remains, for example, about research that presents more than minimal risk without immediate prospect of direct benefit to the children involved. Some have argued that such research is inadmissible, while others have pointed out that this limit would rule out much research promising great benefit to children in the future.

Here again, as with all hard cases, the different claims covered by the principle of beneficence may come into conflict and force difficult choices.

3. Justice

Who ought to receive the benefits of research and bear its burdens? This is a question of justice, in the sense of "fairness in distribution" or "what is deserved." An injustice occurs when some benefit to which a person is entitled is denied without good reason or when some burden is imposed unduly. Another way of conceiving the principle of justice is that equals ought to be treated equally. However, this statement requires explication. Who is equal and who unequal? What considerations justify departure from equal distribution? Almost all commentators allow that distinctions based on experience, age, deprivation, competence, merit and position do sometimes constitute criteria justifying differential treatment for certain purposes. It is necessary, then, to explain in what respects people should be treated equally. There are several widely accepted formulations of just ways to distribute burdens and benefits. Each formulation mentions some relevant property on the basis of which burdens and benefits should be distributed. These formulations are 1) to each person an equal share, 2) to each person according to individual need, 3) to each person according to individual effort, 4) to each person according to societal contribution, and 5) to each person according to merit.

Questions of justice have long been associated with social practices such as punishment, taxation and political representation. Until recently these questions have not generally been associated with scientific research. However, they are foreshadowed even in the earliest reflections on the ethics of research involving human subject. For example, during the 19th and early 20th centuries the burdens of serving as research subjects fell largely upon poor ward patients, while the benefits of improved medical care flowed primarily to private patients. Subsequently, the exploitation of unwilling prisoners as research subjects in Nazi concentration camps was condemned as a particularly flagrant injustice. In this country, in the 1940s, the Tuskegee syphilis study used disadvantaged, rural black men to study the untreated course of a disease that is by no means confined to that population. These subjects were deprived of demonstrably effective treatment in order not to interrupt the project, long after such treatment became generally available.

Against this historical background, it can be seen how conceptions of justice are relevant to research involving human subjects. For example, the selection of research subjects needs to be scrutinized in order to determine whether some classes (e.g., welfare patients, particular racial and ethnic minorities, or persons confined to institutions) are being systematically selected simply because of their easy availability, their compromised position, or their manipulability, rather than for reasons directly related to the problem being studied. Finally, whenever research supported by public funds leads to the development of therapeutic devices and procedures, justice demands both that these not provide advantages only to those who can afford them and that such research should not unduly involve persons from groups unlikely to be among the beneficiaries of subsequent applications of the research.

C. Applications

Application of the general principles to the conduct of research leads to consideration of the following requirements: informed consent, risk/benefit assessment, and the selection of subjects of research.

1. Informed Consent

Respect for persons requires that subjects, to the degree that they care capable, be given the opportunity to choose what shall or shall not happen to them. This opportunity is provided when adequate standards for informed consent are satisfied.

While the importance of informed consent is unquestioned, controversy prevails over the nature and possibility of an informed consent. Nonetheless, there is widespread agreement that the consent process can be analyzed as containing three elements: information, comprehension and voluntariness.

A special problem of consent arises where informing subjects of some pertinent aspect of the research is likely to impair the validity of the research. In many cases it is sufficient to indicate to subjects that they are being invited to participate in research of which some features will not be revealed until the research is concluded. In all cases of research involving incomplete disclosure, such research is justified only if it is clear that 1) incomplete disclosure is truly necessary to accomplish the goals of the research, 2) there are no undisclosed risks to subjects that are more than minimal, and 3) there is an adequate plan for debriefing subjects, when appropriate, and for dissemination of research results to them. Information about risks should never be withheld for the purpose of eliciting the cooperation of subjects, and truthful answers should always be given to direct questions about the research. Care should be taken to distinguish cases in which disclosure would destroy or invalidate the research from cases in which disclosure would simply inconvenience the investigator.

Comprehension. The manner and context in which information is conveyed is as important as the information itself. For example, presenting information in a disorganized and rapid fashion, allowing too little time for consideration or curtailing opportunities for questioning, all may adversely affect a subject's ability to make an informed choice.

Because the subject's ability to understand is a function of intelligence, rationality, maturity and language, it is necessary to adapt the presentation of the information to the subject's capacities. Investigators are responsible for ascertaining that the subject has comprehended the information. While there is always an obligation to ascertain that the information about risk to subjects is complete and adequately comprehended, when the risks are more serious, that obligation increases. On occasion, it may be suitable to give some oral or written test of comprehension.

Special provision may need to be made when comprehension is severely limited--for example, by conditions of immaturity or mental disability. Each class of subjects that one might consider as incompetent (e.g., infants and young children, mentally disabled patients, the terminally ill and the comatose) should be considered on its own terms. Even for these persons, however, respect requires giving them the opportunity to choose to the extent they are able, whether or not to participate in research. The objections of these subjects to involvement should be honored, unless the research entails providing them a therapy unavailable elsewhere. Respect for persons also requires seeking the permission of other parties in order to protect the subjects from harm. Such persons are thus respected both by acknowledging their own wishes and by the use of third parties to protect them from harm.

The third parties chosen should be those who are most likely to understand the incompetent subject's situation and to act in that person's best interest. The person authorized to act on behalf of the subject should be given an opportunity to observe the research as it proceeds in order to be able to withdraw the subject from the research, if such action appears in the subject's best interest.

Voluntariness. An agreement to participate in research constitutes a valid consent only if voluntarily given. This element of informed consent requires conditions free of coercion and undue influence. Coercion occurs when an overt threat of harm is intentionally presented by one person to another in order to obtain compliance. Undue influence, by contrast, occurs through an offer of an excessive, unwarranted, inappropriate or improper reward or other overture in order to obtain compliance. Also, inducements that would ordinarily be acceptable may become undue influences if the subject is especially vulnerable.

Unjustifiable pressures usually occur when persons in positions of authority or commanding influence--especially where possible sanctions are involved--urge a course of action for a subject. A continuum of such influencing factors exists, however, and it is impossible to state precisely where justifiable persuasion ends and undue influence begins. But undue influence would include actions such as manipulating a person's choice through the controlling influence of a close relative and threatening to withdraw health services to which an individual would otherwise be entitled.

2. Assessment of Risks and Benefits

The assessment of risks and benefits requires a careful arrayal of relevant data, including, in some cases, alternative ways of obtaining the benefits sought in the research. Thus, the assessment presents both an opportunity and a responsibility to gather systematic and comprehensive information about proposed research. For the investigator, it is a means to examine whether the proposed research is properly designed. For a review committee, it is a method for determining whether the risks that will be presented to subjects are justified. For prospective subjects, the assessment will assist the determination whether or not to participate.

The nature and scope of risks and benefits. The requirement that research be justified on the basis of a favorable risk/benefit assessment bears a close relation to the principle of beneficence, just as the moral requirement that informed consent be obtained is derived primarily from the principle of respect for persons. The term "risk" refers to a possibility that harm may occur. However, when expressions such as "small risk" or "high risk" are used, they usually refer (often ambiguously) both to the chance (probability) of experiencing a harm and the severity (magnitude) of the envisioned harm.

The term "benefit" is used in the research context to refer to something of positive value related to health or welfare. Unlike "risk," "benefit" is not a term that expresses probabilities. Risk is properly contrasted to probability of benefits, and benefits are properly contrasted with harms rather than risks of harm. Accordingly, so-called risk/benefit assessments are concerned with the probabilities and magnitudes of possible harm and anticipated benefits. Many kinds of possible harms and benefits need be taken into account. There are, for example, risks of psychological harm, physical harm, legal harm, social harm and economic harm and the corresponding benefits. While the most likely types of harms to research subjects are those of psychological or physical pain or injury, other possible kinds should not be overlooked.

Risks and benefits of research may affect the individual subjects, the families of the individual subjects, and society at large (or special groups of subjects in society). Previous codes and federal regulations have required that risks to subjects be outweighed by the sum of both the anticipated benefit to the subject, if any, and the anticipated benefit to society in the form of the knowledge to be gained from the research. In balancing these different elements, the risks and benefits affecting the immediate research subject will normally carry special weight. On the other hand, interests other than those of the subject may on some occasions be sufficient by themselves to justify the risks involved in the research, so long as the subject's rights have been protected. Beneficence thus requires that we protect against risk of harm to subjects and also that we be concerned about the loss of the substantial benefits that might be gained from research.

The systematic assessment of risks and benefits. It is commonly said that benefits and risks must be "balanced" and shown to be "in a favorable ratio." The metaphorical character of these terms draws attention to the difficulty of making precise judgments. Only on rare occasions will quantitative techniques be available for the scrutiny of research protocols. However, the idea of systematic, nonarbitrary analysis of risks and benefits should be emulated insofar as possible. This ideal requires those making decisions about the justifiability of research to be thorough in the accumulation and assessment of information about all aspects of the research, and to consider alternatives systematically. This procedure renders the assessment of research more rigorous and precise, while making communication between review board members and investigators less subject to misinterpretation, misinformation and conflicting judgments. Thus, there should first be a determination of the validity of the presuppositions of the research; then the nature, probability and magnitude of risk should be distinguished with as much clarity as possible. The method of ascertaining risks should be explicit, especially where there is no alternative to the use of such vague categories as small or slight risk. It should also be determined whether an investigator's estimates of the probability of harm or benefits are reasonable, as judged by known facts or other available studies.

Finally, assessment of the justifiability of research should reflect at least the following considerations: (i) Brutal or inhumane treatment of human subjects is never morally justified. (ii) Risks should be reduced to those necessary to achieve the research objective. It should be determined whether it is in fact necessary to use human subjects at all. Risk can perhaps never be entirely eliminated, but it can often be reduced by careful attention to alternative procedures. (iii) When research involves significant risk of serious impairment, review committees should be extraordinarily insistent on the justification of the risk (looking usually to the likelihood of benefit to the subject--or, in some rare cases, to the manifest voluntariness of the participation). (iv) When vulnerable populations are involved in research, the appropriateness of involving them should itself be demonstrated. A number of variables go into such judgments, including the nature and degree of risk, the condition of the particular population involved, and the nature and level of the anticipated benefits. (v) Relevant risks and benefits must be thoroughly arrayed in documents and procedures used in the informed consent process.

3. Selection of Subjects

Just as the principle of respect for persons finds expression in the requirements for consent, and the principle of beneficence in risk/benefit assessment, the principle of justice gives rise to moral requirements that there be fair procedures and outcomes in the selection of research subjects.

Justice is relevant to the selection of subjects of research at two levels: the social and the individual. Individual justice in the selection of subjects would require that researchers exhibit fairness: thus, they should not offer potentially beneficial research to some patients who are in their favor or select only "undesirable" persons for risky research. Social justice requires that a distinction be drawn between classes of subjects that ought, and ought not, to participate in any particular kind of research, based on the ability of members of that class to bear burdens and on the appropriateness of placing further burdens on already burdened persons. Thus, it can be considered a matter of social justice that there is an order of preference in the selection of classes of subjects (e.g., adults before children) and that some classes of potential subjects (e.g., the institutionalized mentally infirm or prisoners) may be involved as research subjects, if at all, only on certain conditions.

Injustice may appear in the selection of subjects, even if individual subjects are selected fairly by investigators and treated fairly in the course of the research. This injustice arises from social, racial, sexual and cultural biases institutionalized in society. Thus, even if individual researchers are treating their research subjects fairly, and even if IRBs are taking care to assure that subjects are selected fairly within a particular institution, unjust social patterns may nevertheless appear in the overall distribution of the burdens and benefits of research. Although individual institutions or investigators may not be able to resolve a problem that is pervasive in their social setting, they can consider distributive justice in selecting research subjects.

Some populations, especially institutionalized ones, are already burdened in many ways by their infirmities and environments. When research is proposed that involves risks and does not include a therapeutic component, other less burdened classes of persons should be called upon first to accept these risks of research, except where the research is directly related to the specific conditions of the class involved. Also, even though public funds for research may often flow in the same directions as public funds for health care, it seems unfair that populations dependent on public health care constitute a pool of preferred research subjects if more advantaged populations are likely to be the recipients of the benefits.

One special instance of injustice results from the involvement of vulnerable subjects. Certain groups, such as racial minorities, the economically disadvantaged, the very sick, and the institutionalized may continually be sought as research subjects, owing to their ready availability in settings where research is conducted. Given their dependent status and their frequently compromised capacity for free consent, they should be protected against the danger of being involved in research solely for administrative convenience, or because they are easy to manipulate as a result of their illness or socioeconomic condition.

Appendices

Appendix A

45 CFR 46: The Federal Regulations Governing Human Experimentation

PART 46--PROTECTION OF HUMAN SUBJECTS

Subpart A--Basic HHS Policy for Protection of Human Research Subjects

Sec.
- 46.101 To what do these regulations apply?
- 46.102 Definitions.
- 46.103 Assurances.
- 46.104 Section reserved.
- 46.105 Section reserved.
- 46.106 Section reserved.
- 46.107 IRB membership.
- 46.108 IRB functions and operations.
- 46.109 IRB review of research.
- 46.110 Expedited review procedures for certain kinds of research involving no more than minimal risk, and for minor changes in approved research.
- 46.111 Criteria for IRB approval of research.
- 46.112 Review by institution.
- 46.113 Suspension or termination of IRB approval of research.
- 46.114 Cooperative research.
- 46.115 IRB records.
- 46.116 General requirements for informed consent.
- 46.117 Documentation of informed consent.
- 46.118 Applications and proposals lacking definite plans for involvement of human subjects.
- 46.119 Research undertaken without the intention of involving human subjects.
- 46.120 Evaluation and disposition of applications and proposals.
- 46.121 Investigational new drug or device 30-day delay requirement.

46.122 Use of federal funds.
46.123 Early termination of research funding: evaluation of subsequent applications and proposals.
46.124 Conditions.

Subpart B--Additional Protections Pertaining to Research, Development, and Related Activities Involving Fetuses, Pregnant Women, and Human In Vitro Fertilization

Sec.
46.201 Applicability.
46.202 Purpose.
46.203 Definitions.
46.204 Ethical Advisory Boards.
46.205 Additional duties of the Institutional Review Boards in connection with activities involving fetuses, pregnant women, or human in vitro fertilization.
46.206 General limitations.
46.207 Activities directed toward pregnant women as subjects.
46.208 Activities directed toward fetuses in utero as subjects.
46.209 Activities directed toward fetuses ex utero, including nonviable fetuses, as subjects.
46.210 Activities involving the dead fetus, fetal material, or the placenta.
46.211 Modification or waiver of specific requirements.

Subpart C--Additional Protections Pertaining to Biomedical and Behavioral Research Involving Prisoners as Subjects

Sec.
46.301 Applicability.
46.302 Purpose.
46.303 Definitions.
46.304 Composition of Institutional Review Boards where prisoners are involved.
46.305 Additional duties of the Institutional Review Boards where prisoners are involved.
46.306 Permitted activities involving prisoners.

Subpart D--Additional Protections for Children Involved as Subjects in Research

Sec.
46.401 To what do these regulations apply?

46.402 Definitions.
46.403 IRB duties.
46.404 Research not involving greater than minimal risk.
46.405 Research involving greater than minimal risk but presenting the prospect of direct benefit to the individual subjects.
46.406 Research involving greater than minimal risk and no prospect of direct benefit to individual subjects, but likely to yield generalizable knowledge about the subject's disorder or condition.
46.407 Research not otherwise approvable which presents an opportunity to understand, prevent, or alleviate a serious problem affecting the health or welfare of children.
46.408 Requirements for permission by parents or guardians and for assent by children.
46.409 Wards.

Authority: 5 U.S.C. 301; sec. 474(a), 88 Stat. 352 (42 U.S.C. 289*l*-3(a)).

Subpart A--Basic HHS Policy for Protection of Human Research Subjects
Source: 46 FR 8386, January 26, 1981, 48 FR 9269, March 4, 1983.

Section 46.101 To what do these regulations apply?

(a) Except as provided in paragraph (b) of this section, this subpart applies to all research involving human subjects conducted by the Department of Health and Human Services or funded in whole or in part by a Department grant, contract, cooperative agreement or fellowship.

(1) This includes research conducted by Department employees, except each Principal Operating Component head may adopt such nonsubstantive, procedural modifications as may be appropriate from an administrative standpoint.

(2) It also includes research conducted or funded by the Department of Health and Human Services outside the United States, but in appropriate circumstances, the Secretary may, under paragraph (e) of this section waive the applicability of some or all of the requirements of these regulations for research of this type.

(b) Research activities in which the only involvement of human subjects will be in one or more of the following categories are exempt from these regulations unless the research is covered by other subparts of this part:

(1) Research conducted in established or commonly accepted educational settings, involving normal educational practices, such as (i) research on regular and special education instructional strategies, or (ii) research on the effectiveness of or the comparison among instructional techniques, curricula, or classroom management methods.

(2) Research involving the use of educational tests (cognitive, diagnostic, aptitude, achievement), if information taken from these sources is recorded in such a manner that subjects cannot be identified, directly or through identifiers linked to the subjects.

(3) Research involving survey or interview procedures, except where all of the following conditions exist: (i) responses are recorded in such a manner that the human subjects can be identified, directly or through identifiers linked to the subjects, (ii) the subject's responses, if they became known outside the research, could reasonably place the subject at risk of criminal or civil liability or be damaging to the subject's financial standing or employability, and (iii) the research deals with sensitive aspects of the subject's own behavior, such as illegal conduct, drug use, sexual behavior, or use of alcohol. All research involving survey or interview procedures is exempt, without exception, when the respondents are elected or appointed public officials or candidates for public office.

(4) Research involving the observation (including observation by participants) of public behavior, except where all of the following conditions exist: (i) observations are recorded in such a manner that the human subjects can be identified, directly or through identifiers linked to the subjects, (ii) the observations recorded about the individual, if they became known outside the research, could reasonably place the subject at risk of criminal or civil liability or be damaging to the subject's financial standing or employability, and (iii) the research deals with sensitive aspects of the subject's own behavior such as illegal conduct, drug use, sexual behavior, or use of alcohol.

(5) Research involving the collection or study of existing data, documents, records, pathological specimens, or diagnostic specimens, if these sources are publicly available or if the information is recorded by the investigator in such a manner that subjects cannot be identified, directly or through identifiers linked to the subjects.

(6) Unless specifically required by statute (and except to the extent specified in paragraph (i)), research and demonstration projects which are conducted by or subject to the approval of the Department of Health and Human Services, and which are designed to study, evaluate, or otherwise examine: (i) programs under the Social Security Act, or other public benefit or service programs; (ii) procedures for obtaining benefits or services under those programs; (iii) possible changes in or alternatives to those programs or procedures; or (iv) possible changes in methods or levels of payment for benefits or services under those programs.

(c) The Secretary has final authority to determine whether a particular activity is covered by these regulations.

(d) The Secretary may require that specific research activities or classes of research activities conducted or funded by the Department, but not otherwise covered by these regulations, comply with some or all of these regulations.

(e) The Secretary may also waive applicability of these regulations to specific research activities or classes of research activities, otherwise covered by these regulations. Notices of these actions will be published in the *Federal Register* as they occur.

(f) No individual may receive Department funding for research covered by these regulations unless the individual is affiliated with or sponsored by an institution which assumes responsibility for the research under an assurance satisfying the requirements of this part, or the individual makes other arrangements with the Department.

(g) Compliance with these regulations will in no way render inapplicable pertinent federal, state, or local laws or regulations.

(h) Each subpart of these regulations contains a separate section describing to what the subpart applies. Research which is covered by more than one subpart shall comply with all applicable subparts.

(i) If, following review of proposed research activities that are exempt from these regulations under paragraph (b)(6), the Secretary determines that a research or demonstration project presents a danger to the physical, mental, or emotional well-being of a participant or subject of the research or demonstration project, then federal funds may not be expended for such a project without the written, informed consent of each participant or subject.

Section 46.102 Definitions.

(a) "Secretary" means the Secretary of Health and Human Services and any other officer or employee of the Department of Health and Human Services to whom authority has been delegated.

(b) "Department" or "HHS" means the Department of Health and Human Services.

(c) "Institution" means any public or private entity or agency (including federal, state, and other agencies).

(d) "Legally authorized representative" means an individual or judicial or other body authorized under applicable law to consent on behalf of a prospective subject to the subject's participation in the procedure(s) involved in the research.

(e) "Research" means a systematic investigation designed to develop or contribute to generalizable knowledge. Activities which meet this definition constitute "research" for purposes of these regulations, whether or not they are supported or funded under a program which is considered research for other purposes. For example, some "demonstration" and "service" programs may include research activities.

(f) "Human subject" means a living individual about whom an investigator (whether professional or student) conducting research obtains (1) data through intervention or interaction with the individual, or (2) identifiable private information. "Intervention" includes both physical procedures by which data are gathered (for example, venipuncture) and manipulations of the subject or the subject's environment that are performed for research purposes. "Interaction" includes communication or interpersonal contact between investigator and subject. "Private information" includes information about behavior that occurs in a context in which an individual can reasonably expect that no observation or recording is taking place, and information which has been provided for specific purposes by an individual and which the individual can reasonably expect will not be made public (for example, a medical record). Private information must be individually identifiable (i.e., the identity of the subject is or may readily be ascertained by the investigator or associated with the information) in order for obtaining the information to constitute research involving human subjects.

(g) "Minimal risk" means that the risks of harm anticipated in the proposed research are not greater, considering probability and magnitude, than those ordinarily encountered in daily life or during the performance of routine physical or psychological examinations or tests.

(h) "Certification" means the official notification by the institution to the Department in accordance with the requirements of this part that a research project or activity involving human subjects has been reviewed and approved by the Institutional Review Board (IRB) in accordance with the approved assurance on file at HHS. (Certification is required when the research is funded by the Department and not otherwise exempt in accordance with section 46.101(b)).

Section 46.103 Assurances.

(a) Each institution engaged in research covered by these regulations shall provide written assurance satisfactory to the Secretary that it will comply with the requirements set forth in these regulations.

(b) The Department will conduct or fund research covered by these regulations only if the institution has an assurance approved as provided in this section, and only if the institution has certified to the Secretary that the research has been reviewed and approved by an IRB provided for in the assurance, and will be subject to continuing review by the IRB. This assurance shall at a minimum include:

(1) A statement of principles governing the institution in the discharge of its responsibilities for protecting the rights and welfare of human subjects of research conducted at or sponsored by the institution, regardless of source of funding. This may include an appropriate existing code, declaration, or statement of ethical principles, or a statement formulated by the institution itself. This requirement does not preempt provisions of these regulations applicable to Department-funded research and is not applicable to any research in an exempt category listed in section 46.101.

(2) Designation of one or more IRBs established in accordance with the requirements of this subpart, and for which provisions are made for meeting space and sufficient staff to support the IRB's review and recordkeeping duties.

(3) A list of the IRB members identified by name; earned degrees; representative capacity; indications of experience such as board certifications, licenses, etc., sufficient to describe each member's chief anticipated contributions to IRB deliberations; and any employment or other relationship between each member and the institution; for example: full-time employee, part-time employee, member of governing panel or board, stockholder, paid or unpaid consultant. Changes in IRB membership shall be reported to the Secretary.[1]

(4) Written procedures which the IRB will follow (i) for conducting its initial and continuing review of research and for reporting its findings and actions to the investigator and the institution; (ii) for determining which projects require review more often than annually and which projects need verification from sources other than the investigators that no material changes have occurred since previous IRB review; (iii) for insuring prompt reporting to the IRB of proposed changes in a research activity, and for insuring that changes in approved research, during the period for which IRB approval has already been given, may not be initiated without IRB review and approval except where necessary to eliminate apparent immediate hazards to the subject; and (iv) for insuring prompt reporting to the IRB and to the Secretary[1] of unanticipated problems involving risks to subjects or others.

(c) The assurance shall be executed by an individual authorized to act for the institution and to assume on behalf of the institution the obligations imposed by these regulations, and shall be filed in such form and manner as the Secretary may prescribe.

(d) The Secretary will evaluate all assurances submitted in accordance with these regulations through such officers and employees of the Department and such experts or consultants engaged for this purpose as the Secretary determines to be appropriate. The Secretary's evaluation will take into consideration the adequacy of the proposed IRB in light of the anticipated scope of the institution's research activities and the types of subject populations likely to be involved, the appropriateness of the proposed initial and continuing review procedures in light of the probable risks, and the size and complexity of the institution.

(e) On the basis of this evaluation, the Secretary may approve or disapprove the assurance, or enter into negotiations to develop an approvable one. The Secretary may limit the period during which any particular approved assurance or class of approved assurances shall remain effective or otherwise condition or restrict approval.

---

[1] Reports should be filed with the Office for Protection from Research Risks, National Institutes of Health, Department of Health and Human Services, Bethesda, Maryland 20205.

(f) Within 60 days after the day of submission to HHS of an application or proposal, an institution with an approved assurance covering the proposed research shall certify that the application or proposal has been reviewed and approved by the IRB. Other institutions shall certify that the application or proposal has been approved by the IRB within 30 days after receipt of a request for such a certification from the Department. If the certification is not submitted within these time limits, the application or proposal may be returned to the institution.

Section 46.104 [Reserved]

Section 46.105 [Reserved]

Section 46.106 [Reserved]

Section 46.107 IRB membership.

(a) Each IRB shall have at least five members, with varying backgrounds to promote complete and adequate review of research activities commonly conducted by the institution. The IRB shall be sufficiently qualified through the experience and expertise of its members, and the diversity of the members' backgrounds including consideration of the racial and cultural backgrounds of members and sensitivity to such issues as community attitudes, to promote respect for its advice and counsel in safeguarding the rights and welfare of human subjects. In addition to possessing the professional competence necessary to review specific research activities, the IRB shall be able to ascertain the acceptability of proposed research in terms of institutional commitments and regulations, applicable law, and standards of professional conduct and practice. The IRB shall therefore include persons knowledgeable in these areas. If an IRB regularly reviews research that involves a vulnerable category of subjects, including but not limited to subjects covered by other subparts of this part, the IRB shall include one or more individuals who are primarily concerned with the welfare of these subjects.

(b) No IRB may consist entirely of men or entirely of women, or entirely of members of one profession.

(c) Each IRB shall include at least one member whose primary concerns are in nonscientific areas; for example; lawyers, ethicists, members of the clergy.

(d) Each IRB shall include at least one member who is not otherwise affiliated with the institution and who is not part of the immediate family of a person who is affiliated with the institution.

(e) No IRB may have a member participating in the IRB's initial or continuing review of any project in which the member has a conflicting interest, except to provide information requested by the IRB.

(f) An IRB may, in its discretion, invite individuals with competence in special areas to assist in the review of complex issues which require expertise beyond or in addition to that available on the IRB. These individuals may not vote with the IRB.

Section 46.108 IRB functions and operations.
In order to fulfill the requirements of these regulations each IRB shall:

(a) Follow written procedures as provided in section 46.103(b)(4).

(b) Except when an expedited review procedure is used (see section 46.110), review proposed research at convened meetings at which a majority of the members of the IRB are present, including at least one member whose primary concerns are in nonscientific areas. In order for the research to be approved, it shall receive the approval of a majority of those members present at the meeting.

(c) Be responsible for reporting to the appropriate institutional officials and the Secretary[1] any serious or continuing noncompliance by investigators with the requirements and determinations of the IRB.

Section 46.109 IRB review of research.

(a) An IRB shall review and have authority to approve, require modifications in (to secure approval), or disapprove all research activities covered by these regulations.

(b) An IRB shall require that information given to subjects as part of informed consent is in accordance with section 46.116. The IRB may require that information, in addition to that specifically mentioned in section 46.116, be given to the subjects when in the IRB's judgment the information would meaningfully add to the protection of the rights and welfare of subjects.

(c) An IRB shall require documentation of informed consent or may waive documentation in accordance with section 46.117.

(d) An IRB shall notify investigators and the institution in writing of its decision to approve or disapprove the proposed research activity, or of modifications required to secure IRB approval of the research activity. If the IRB decides to disapprove a research activity, it shall include in its written notification a statement of the reasons for its decision and give the investigator an opportunity to respond in person or in writing.

(e) An IRB shall conduct continuing review of research covered by these regulations at intervals appropriate to the degree of risk, but not less than once

---

[1] Reports should be filed with the Office for Protection from Research Risks, National Institutes of Health, Department of Health and Human Services, Bethesda, Maryland 20205.

per year, and shall have authority to observe or have a third party observe the consent process and the research.

Section 46.110 Expedited review procedures for certain kinds of research involving no more than minimal risk, and for minor changes in approved research.

(a) The Secretary has established, and published in the *Federal Register*, a list of categories of research that may be reviewed by the IRB through an expedited review procedure. The list will be amended, as appropriate, through periodic republication in the *Federal Register*.

(b) An IRB may review some or all of the research appearing on the list through an expedited review procedure, if the research involves no more than minimal risk. The IRB may also use the expedited review procedure to review minor changes in previously approved research during the period for which approval is authorized. Under an expedited review procedure, the review may be carried out by the IRB chairperson or by one or more experienced reviewers designated by the chairperson from among members of the IRB. In reviewing the research, the reviewers may exercise all of the authorities of the IRB except that the reviewers may not disapprove the research. A research activity may be disapproved only after review in accordance with the non-expedited procedure set forth in section 46.108(b).

(c) Each IRB which uses an expedited review procedure shall adopt a method for keeping all members advised of research proposals which have been approved under the procedure.

(d) The Secretary may restrict, suspend, or terminate an institution's or IRB's use of the expedited review procedure when necessary to protect the rights or welfare of subjects.

Section 46.111 Criteria for IRB approval of research.

(a) In order to approve research covered by these regulations the IRB shall determine that all of the following requirements are satisfied:

(1) Risks to subjects are minimized: (i) By using procedures which are consistent with sound research design and which do not unnecessarily expose subjects to risk, and (ii) whenever appropriate, by using procedures already being performed on the subjects for diagnostic or treatment purposes.

(2) Risks to subjects are reasonable in relation to anticipated benefits, if any, to subjects, and the importance of the knowledge that may reasonably be expected to result. In evaluating risks and benefits, the IRB should consider only those risks and benefits that may result from the research (as distinguished from risks and benefits of therapies subjects would receive even if not participating in the research). The IRB should not consider possible long-range effects of applying knowledge gained in the research (for example, the possible

effects of the research on public policy) as among those research risks that fall within the purview of its responsibility.

(3) Selection of subjects is equitable. In making this assessment the IRB should take into account the purposes of the research and the setting in which the research will be conducted.

(4) Informed consent will be sought from each prospective subject or the subject's legally authorized representative, in accordance with, and to the extent required by section 46.116.

(5) Informed consent will be appropriately documented, in accordance with, and to the extent required by section 46.117.

(6) Where appropriate, the research plan makes adequate provision for monitoring the data collected to insure the safety of subjects.

(7) Where appropriate, there are adequate provisions to protect the privacy of subjects and to maintain the confidentiality of data.

(b) Where some or all of the subjects are likely to be vulnerable to coercion or undue influence, such as persons with acute or severe physical or mental illness, or persons who are economically or educationally disadvantaged, appropriate additional safeguards have been included in the study to protect the rights and welfare of these subjects.

Section 46.112 Review by institution.

Research covered by these regulations that has been approved by an IRB may be subject to further appropriate review and approval or disapproval by officials of the institution. However, those officials may not approve the research if it has not been approved by an IRB.

Section 46.113 Suspension or termination of IRB approval of research.

An IRB shall have authority to suspend or terminate approval of research that is not being conducted in accordance with the IRB's requirements or that has been associated with unexpected serious harm to subjects. Any suspension or termination of approval shall include a statement of the reasons for the IRB's action and shall be reported promptly to the investigator, appropriate institutional officials, and the Secretary.[1]

Section 46.114 Cooperative research.

Cooperative research projects are those projects, normally supported through grants, contracts, or similar arrangements, which involve institutions in addition to the grantee or prime contractor (such as a contractor with the grantee, or a subcontractor with the prime contractor). In such instances, the grantee or prime contractor remains responsible to the Department for safe-

---

[1] Reports should be filed with the Office for Protection from Research Risks, National Institutes of Health, Department of Health and Human Services, Bethesda, Maryland 20205.

guarding the rights and welfare of human subjects. Also, when cooperating institutions conduct some or all of the research involving some or all of these subjects, each cooperating institution shall comply with these regulations as though it received funds for its participation in the project directly from the Department, except that in complying with these regulations institutions may use joint review, reliance upon the review of another qualified IRB, or similar arrangements aimed at avoidance of duplication of effort.

Section 46.115 IRB records.

(a) An institution, or where appropriate an IRB, shall prepare and maintain adequate documentation of IRB activities, including the following:

(1) Copies of all research proposals reviewed, scientific evaluations, if any, that accompany the proposals, approved sample consent documents, progress reports submitted by investigators, and reports of injuries to subjects.

(2) Minutes of IRB meetings which shall be in sufficient detail to show attendance at the meetings; actions taken by the IRB; the vote on these actions including the number of members voting for, against, and abstaining; the basis for requiring changes in or disapproving research; and a written summary of the discussion of controverted issues and their resolution.

(3) Records of continuing review activities.

(4) Copies of all correspondence between the IRB and the investigators.

(5) A list of IRB members as required by section 46.103(b)(3).

(6) Written procedures for the IRB as required by section 46.103(b)(4).

(7) Statements of significant new findings provided to subjects, as required by section 46.116(b)(5).

(b) The records required by this regulation shall be retained for at least 3 years after completion of the research, and the records shall be accessible for inspection and copying by authorized representatives of the Department at reasonable times and in a reasonable manner.

Section 46.116 General requirements for informed consent.

Except as provided elsewhere in this or other subparts, no investigator may involve a human being as a subject in research covered by these regulations unless the investigator has obtained the legally effective informed consent of the subject or the subject's legally authorized representative. An investigator shall seek such consent only under circumstances that provide the prospective subject or the representative sufficient opportunity to consider whether or not to participate and that minimize the possibility of coercion or undue influence. The information that is given to the subject or the representative shall be in language understandable to the subject or the representative. No informed consent, whether oral or written, may include any exculpatory language through which the subject or the representative is made to waive or appear to waive any of the subject's legal rights, or releases or appears to release the investigator, the sponsor, the institution or its agents from liability for negligence.

(a) Basic elements of informed consent. Except as provided in paragraph (c) or (d) of this section, in seeking informed consent the following information shall be provided to each subject:

(1) A statement that the study involves research, an explanation of the purposes of the research and the expected duration of the subject's participation, a description of the procedures to be followed, and identification of any procedures which are experimental;

(2) A description of any reasonably foreseeable risks or discomforts to the subject;

(3) A description of any benefits to the subject or to others which may reasonably be expected from the research;

(4) A disclosure of appropriate alternative procedures or courses of treatment, if any, that might be advantageous to the subject;

(5) A statement describing the extent, if any, to which confidentiality of records identifying the subject will be maintained;

(6) For research involving more than minimal risk, an explanation as to whether any compensation and an explanation as to whether any medical treatments are available if injury occurs and, if so, what they consist of, or where further information may be obtained;

(7) An explanation of whom to contact for answers to pertinent questions about the research and research subjects' rights, and whom to contact in the event of a research-related injury to the subject; and

(8) A statement that participation is voluntary, refusal to participate will involve no penalty or loss of benefits to which the subject is otherwise entitled, and the subject may discontinue participation at any time without penalty or loss of benefits to which the subject is otherwise entitled.

(b) Additional elements of informed consent. When appropriate, one or more of the following elements of information shall also be provided to each subject:

(1) A statement that the particular treatment or procedure may involve risks to the subject (or to the embryo or fetus, if the subject is or may become pregnant) which are currently unforeseeable;

(2) Anticipated circumstances under which the subject's participation may be terminated by the investigator without regard to the subject's consent;

(3) Any additional costs to the subject that may result from participation in the research;

(4) The consequences of a subject's decision to withdraw from the research and procedures for orderly termination of participation by the subject;

(5) A statement that significant new findings developed during the course of the research which may relate to the subject's willingness to continue participation will be provided to the subject; and

(6) The approximate number of subjects involved in the study.

(c) An IRB may approve a consent procedure which does not include, or which alters, some or all of the elements of informed consent set forth above, or waive the requirement to obtain informed consent provided the IRB finds and documents that:

(1) The research or demonstration project is to be conducted by or subject to the approval of state or local government officials and is designed to study, evaluate, or otherwise examine: (i) programs under the Social Security Act, or other public benefit or service programs, (ii) procedures for obtaining benefits or services under those programs; (iii) possible changes in or alternatives to those programs or procedures; or (iv) possible changes in methods or levels of payment for benefits or services under those programs; and

(2) The research could not practicably be carried out without the waiver or alteration.

(d) An IRB may approve a consent procedure which does not include, or which alters, some or all of the elements of informed consent set forth above, or waive the requirements to obtain informed consent provided the IRB finds and documents that:

(1) The research involves no more than minimal risk to the subjects;

(2) The waiver or alteration will not adversely affect the rights and welfare of the subjects;

(3) The research could not practicably be carried out without the waiver or alteration; and

(4) Whenever appropriate, the subjects will be provided with additional pertinent information after participation.

(e) The informed consent requirements in these regulations are not intended to preempt any applicable federal, state, or local laws which require additional information to be disclosed in order for informed consent to be legally effective.

(f) Nothing in these regulations is intended to limit the authority of a physician to provide emergency medical care, to the extent the physician is permitted to do so under applicable federal, state, or local law.

Section 46.117 Documentation of informed consent.

(a) Except as provided in paragraph (c) of this section, informed consent shall be documented by the use of a written consent form approved by the IRB and signed by the subject or the subject's legally authorized representative. A copy shall be given to the person signing the form.

(b) Except as provided in paragraph (c) of this section, the consent form may be either of the following:

(1) A written consent document that embodies the elements of informed consent required by section 46.116. This form may be read to the subject or the subject's legally authorized representative, but in any event, the investigator

shall give either the subject or the representative adequate opportunity to read it before it is signed; or

(2) A "short form" written consent document stating that the elements of informed consent required by section 46.116 have been presented orally to the subject or the subject's legally authorized representative. When this method is used, there shall be a witness to the oral presentation. Also, the IRB shall approve a written summary of what is to be said to the subject or the representative. Only the short form itself is to be signed by the subject or the representative. However, the witness shall sign both the short form and a copy of the summary, and the person actually obtaining consent shall sign a copy of the summary. A copy of the summary shall be given to the subject or the representative, in addition to a copy of the "short form."

(c) An IRB may waive the requirement for the investigator to obtain a signed consent form for some or all subjects if it finds either:

(1) That the only record linking the subject and the research would be the consent document and the principal risk would be potential harm resulting from a breach of confidentiality. Each subject will be asked whether the subject wants documentation linking the subject with the research, and the subject's wishes will govern; or

(2) That the research presents no more than minimal risk of harm to subjects and involves no procedures for which written consent is normally required outside of the research context.

In cases where the documentation requirement is waived, the IRB may require the investigator to provide subjects with a written statement regarding the research.

Section 46.118 Applications and proposals lacking definite plans for involvement of human subjects.

Certain types of applications for grants, cooperative agreements, or contracts are submitted to the Department with the knowledge that subjects may be involved within the period of funding, but definite plans would not normally be set forth in the application of proposal. These include activities such as institutional type grants (including bloc grants) where selection of specific projects is the institution's responsibility; research training grants where the activities involving subjects remain to be selected; and projects in which human subjects' involvement will depend upon completion of instruments, prior animal studies, or purification of compounds. These applications need not be reviewed by an IRB before an award may be made. However, except for research described in section 46.101(b), no human subjects may be involved in any project supported by these awards until the project has been reviewed and approved by the IRB, as provided in these regulations, and certification submitted to the Department.

Section 46.119 Research undertaken without the intention of involving human subjects.

In the event research (conducted or funded by the Department) is undertaken without the intention of involving human subjects, but it is later proposed to use human subjects in the research, the research shall first be reviewed and approved by an IRB, as provided in these regulations, a certification submitted to the Department, and final approval given to the proposed change by the Department.

Section 46.120 Evaluation and disposition of applications and proposals.

(a) The Secretary will evaluate all applications and proposals involving human subjects submitted to the Department through such officers and employees of the Department and such experts and consultants as the Secretary determines to be appropriate. This evaluation will take into consideration the risks to the subjects, the adequacy of protection against these risks, the potential benefits of the proposed research to the subjects and others, and the importance of the knowledge to be gained.

(b) On the basis of this evaluation, the Secretary may approve or disapprove the application or proposal, or enter into negotiations to develop an approvable one.

Section 46.121 Investigational new drug or device 30-day delay requirement.

When an institution is required to prepare or to submit a certification with an application or proposal under these regulations, and the application or proposal involves an investigational new drug (within the meaning of 21 U.S.C. 355(i) or 357(d)) or a significant risk device (as defined in 21 CFR 812.3(m)), the institution shall identify the drug or device in the certification. The institution shall also state whether the 30-day interval required for investigational new drugs by 21 CFR 312.1(a) and for significant risk devices by 21 CFR 812.30 has elapsed, or whether the Food and Drug Administration has waived that requirement. If the 30-day interval has expired, the institution shall state whether the Food and Drug Administration has requested that the sponsor continue to withhold or restrict the use of the drug or device in human subjects. If the 30-day interval has not expired, and a waiver has not been received, the institution shall send a statement to the Department upon expiration of the interval. The Department will not consider a certification acceptable until the institution has submitted a statement that the 30-day interval has elapsed, and the Food and Drug Administration has not requested it to limit the use of the drug or device, or that the Food and Drug Administration has waived the 30-day interval.

Section 46.122 Use of Federal funds.

Federal funds administered by the Department may not be expended for research involving human subjects unless the requirement of these regulations, including all subparts of these regulations, have been satisfied.

Section 46.123 Early termination of research funding; evaluation of subsequent applications and proposals.

(a) The Secretary may require that Department funding for any project be terminated or suspended in the manner prescribed in applicable program requirements, when the Secretary finds an institution has materially failed to comply with the terms of these regulations.

(b) In making decisions about funding applications or proposals covered by these regulations the Secretary may take into account, in addition to all other eligibility requirements and program criteria, factors such as whether the applicant has been subject to a termination or suspension under paragraph (a) of this section and whether the applicant or the person who would direct the scientific and technical aspects of an activity has in the judgment of the Secretary materially failed to discharge responsibility for the protection of the rights and welfare of human subjects (whether or not Department funds were involved).

Section 46.124 Conditions.

With respect to any research project or any class of research projects the Secretary may impose additional conditions prior to or at the time of funding when in the Secretary's judgment additional conditions are necessary for the protection of human subjects.

Subpart B--Additional Protections Pertaining to Research Development, and Related Activities Involving Fetuses, Pregnant Women, and Human in Vitro Fertilization.

Source: 40 FR 33528, Aug. 8, 1975, 43 FR 1758, January 11, 1978, 43 FR 51559, November 3, 1978.

Section 46.201 Applicability.

(a) The regulations in this subpart are applicable to all Department of Health, Education, and Welfare grants and contract supporting research, development, and related activities involving: (1) The fetus, (2) pregnant women, and (3) human *in vitro* fertilization.

(b) Nothing in this subpart shall be construed as indicating that compliance with the procedures set forth herein will in any way render inapplicable pertinent State or local laws bearing upon activities covered by this subpart.

(c) The requirements of this subpart are in addition to those imposed under the other subparts of this part.

Section 46.202 Purpose.

It is the purpose of this subpart to provide additional safeguards in reviewing activities to which this subpart is applicable to assure that they conform to appropriate ethical standards and relate to important societal needs.

Section 46.203 Definitions.

As used in this subpart:

(a) "Secretary" means the Secretary of Health and Human Services and any other officer or employee of the Department of Health and Human Services to whom authority has been delegated.

(b) "Pregnancy" encompasses the period of time from confirmation of implantation (through any of the presumptive signs of pregnancy, such as missed menses, or by a medically acceptable pregnancy test), until expulsion or extraction of the fetus.

(c) "Fetus" means the product of conception from the time of implantation (as evidenced by any of the presumptive signs of pregnancy, such as missed menses, or a medically acceptable pregnancy test), until a determination is made, following expulsion or extraction of the fetus, that it is viable.

(d) "Viable" as it pertains to the fetus means being able, after either spontaneous or induced delivery, to survive (given the benefit of available medical therapy) to the point of independently maintaining heart beat and respiration. The Secretary may from time to time, taking into account medical advances, publish in the *Federal Register* guidelines to assist in determining whether a fetus is viable for purposes of this subpart. If a fetus is viable after delivery, it is a premature infant.

(e) "Nonviable fetus" means a fetus *ex utero* which, although living, is not viable.

(f) "Dead fetus" means a fetus *ex utero* which exhibits neither heartbeat, spontaneous respiratory activity, spontaneous movement of voluntary muscles, nor pulsation of the umbilical cord (if still attached).

(g) "*In vitro* fertilization" means any fertilization of human ova which occurs outside the body of a female, either through admixture of donor human sperm and ova or by any other means.

Section 46.204 Ethical Advisory Boards.

(a) One or more Ethical Advisory Boards shall be established by the Secretary. Members of these board(s) shall be so selected that the board(s) will be competent to deal with medical, legal, social, ethical, and related issues and may include, for example, research scientists, physicians, psychologists, sociologists, educators, lawyers, and ethicists, as well as representatives of the general public. No board member may be a regular, full-time employee of the Department of Health and Human Services.

(b) At the request of the Secretary, the Ethical Advisory Board shall render advice consistent with the policies and requirements of this part as to ethical issues, involving activities covered by this subpart, raised by individual applications or proposals. In addition, upon request by the Secretary, the Board shall render advice as to classes of applications or proposals and general policies, guidelines, and procedures.

(c) A Board may establish, with the approval of the Secretary, classes of applications or proposals which: (1) Must be submitted to the Board, or (2) need not be submitted to the Board. Where the Board so establishes a class of applications or proposals which must be submitted, no application or proposal within the class may be funded by the Department or any component thereof until the application or proposal has been reviewed by the Board and the Board has rendered advice as to its acceptability from an ethical standpoint.

(d) No application or proposal involving human *in vitro* fertilization may be funded by the Department or any component thereof until the application or proposal has been reviewed by the Ethical Advisory Board and the Board has rendered advice as to its acceptability from an ethical standpoint.

Section 46.205 Additional duties of the Institutional Review Boards in connection with activities involving fetuses, pregnant women, or human in vitro fertilization.

(a) In addition to the responsibilities prescribed for Institutional Review Boards under Subpart A of this part, the applicant's or offeror's Board shall, with respect to activities covered by this subpart, carry out the following additional duties:

(1) Determine that all aspects of the activity meet the requirements of this subpart;

(2) Determine that adequate consideration has been given to the manner in which potential subjects will be selected, and adequate provision has been made by the applicant or offeror for monitoring the actual informed consent process (e.g., through such mechanisms, when appropriate, as participation by the Institutional Review Board or subject advocates in: (i) Overseeing the actual process by which individual consents required by this subpart are secured either by approving induction of each individual into the activity or verifying, perhaps through sampling, that approved procedures for induction of the individuals into the activity are being followed, and (ii) monitoring the progress of the activity and intervening as necessary through such steps as visits to the activity site and continuing evaluation to determine if any unanticipated risks have arisen);

(3) Carry out such other responsibilities as may be assigned by the Secretary.

(b) No award may be issued until the applicant or offeror has certified to the Secretary that the Institutional Review Board has made the determinations required under paragraph (a) of this section and the Secretary has approved these determinations, as provided in Section 46.120 of Subpart A of this part.

(c) Applicants or offerors seeking support for activities covered by this subpart must provide for the designation of an Institutional Review Board, subject to approval by the Secretary, where no such Board has been established under Subpart A of this part.

Section 46.206 General limitations.

(a) No activity to which this subpart is applicable may be undertaken unless:

(1) Appropriate studies on animals and nonpregnant individuals have been completed;

(2) Except where the purpose of the activity is to meet the health needs of the mother or the particular fetus, the risk to the fetus is minimal and, in all cases, is the least possible risk for achieving the objectives of the activity.

(3) Individuals engaged in the activity will have no part in: (i) Any decisions as to the timing, method, and procedures used to terminate the pregnancy, and (ii) determining the viability of the fetus at the termination of the pregnancy; and

(4) No procedural changes which may cause greater than minimal risk to the fetus or the pregnant woman will be introduced into the procedure for terminating the pregnancy solely in the interest of the activity.

(b) No inducements, monetary or otherwise, may be offered to terminate pregnancy for purposes of the activity.

[40 FR 33528, Aug. 8, 1975, as amended at 40 FR 51638, Nov. 6, 1975]

Section 46.207 Activities directed toward pregnant women as subjects.

(a) No pregnant woman may be involved as a subject in an activity covered by this subpart unless: (1) The purpose of the activity is to meet the health needs of the mother and the fetus will be placed at risk only to the minimum extent necessary to meet such needs, or (2) the risk to the fetus is minimal.

(b) An activity permitted under paragraph (a) of this section may be conducted only if the mother and father are legally competent and have given their informed consent after having been fully informed regarding possible impact on the fetus, except that the father's informed consent need not be secured if: (1) The purpose of the activity is to meet the health needs of the mother; (2) his identity or whereabouts cannot reasonably be ascertained; (3) he is not reasonably available; or (4) the pregnancy resulted from rape.

Section 46.208 Activities directed toward fetuses in utero as subjects.

(a) No fetus *in utero* may be involved as a subject in any activity covered by this subpart unless: (1) The purpose of the activity is to meet the health needs of the particular fetus and the fetus will be placed at risk only to the minimum extent necessary to meet such needs, or (2) the risk to the fetus imposed by the research is minimal and the purpose of the activity is the development of important biomedical knowledge which cannot be obtained by other means.

(b) An activity permitted under paragraph (a) of this section may be conducted only if the mother and father are legally competent and have given their informed consent, except that the father's consent need not be secured if: (1) His identity or whereabouts cannot reasonably be ascertained, (2) he is not reasonably available, or (3) the pregnancy resulted from rape.

Section 46.209 Activities directed toward fetuses ex utero, including nonviable fetuses, as subjects.

(a) Until it has been ascertained whether or not a fetus *ex utero* is viable, a fetus ex utero may not be involved as a subject in an activity covered by this subpart unless:

(1) There will be no added risk to the fetus resulting from the activity, and the purpose of the activity is the development of important biomedical knowledge which cannot be obtained by other means, or

(2) The purpose of the activity is to enhance the possibility of survival of the particular fetus to the point of viability.

(b) No nonviable fetus may be involved as a subject in an activity covered by this subpart unless:

(1) Vital functions of the fetus will not be artificially maintained,

(2) Experimental activities which of themselves would terminate the heartbeat or respiration of the fetus will not be employed, and

(3) The purpose of the activity is the development of important biomedical knowledge which cannot be obtained by other means.

(c) In the event the fetus *ex utero* is found to be viable, it may be included as a subject in the activity only to the extent permitted by and in accordance with requirements of other subparts of this part.

(d) An activity permitted under paragraph (a) or (b) of this section may be conducted only if the mother and father are legally competent and have given their informed consent, except that the father's informed consent need not be secured if: (1) his identify or whereabouts cannot reasonably be ascertained, (2) he is not reasonably available, or (3) the pregnancy resulted from rape.

Section 46.210 Activities involving the dead fetus, fetal material, or the placenta.

Activities involving the dead fetus, macerated fetal material, or cells, tissue, or organs excised from a dead fetus shall be conducted only in accordance with any applicable State or local laws regarding such activities.

Section 46.211 Modifications or waiver of specific requirements.

Upon the request of an applicant or offeror (with the approval of its Institutional Review Board), the Secretary may modify or waive specific requirements of this subpart, with the approval of the Ethical Advisory Board after such opportunity for public comments as the Ethical Advisory Board considers appropriate in the particular instance. In making such decisions, the Secretary will consider whether the risks to the subject are so outweighed by the sum of the benefit to the subject and the importance of the knowledge to be gained as to warrant such modification or waiver and that such benefits cannot be gained except through a modification or waiver. Any such modifications or waivers will be published as notices in the *Federal Register*.

Subpart C--Additional Protections Pertaining to Biomedical and Behavioral Research Involving Prisoners as Subjects
Source: 43 FR 53655, Nov. 16, 1978.

Section 46.301 Applicability.

(a) The regulations in this subpart are applicable to all biomedical and behavioral research conducted or supported by the Department of Health and Human Services involving prisoners as subjects.

(b) Nothing in this subpart shall be construed as indicating that compliance with the procedures set forth herein will authorize research involving prisoners as subjects, to the extent such research is limited or barred by applicable State or local law.

(c) The requirements of this subpart are in addition to those imposed under the other subparts of this part.

Section 46.302 Purpose.

Inasmuch as prisoners may be under constraints because of their incarceration which could affect their ability to make a truly voluntary and uncoerced decision whether or not to participate as subjects in research, it is the purpose of this subpart to provide additional safeguards for the protection of prisoners involved in activities to which this subpart is applicable.

Section 46.303 Definitions.

As used in this subpart:

(a) "Secretary" means the Secretary of Health and Human Services and any other officer or employee of the Department of Health and Human Services to whom authority has been delegated.

(b) "DHHS" means the Department of Health and Human Services.

(c) "Prisoner" means any individual involuntarily confined or detained in a penal institution. The term is intended to encompass individuals sentenced to such an institution under a criminal or civil statute, individuals detained in other facilities by virtue of statutes or commitment procedures which provide alternatives to criminal prosecution or incarceration in a penal institution, and individuals detained pending arraignment, trial, or sentencing.

(d) "Minimal risk" is the probability and magnitude of physical or psychological harm that is normally encountered in the daily lives, or in the routine medical, dental, or psychological examination of healthy persons.

Section 46.304 Composition of Institutional Review Boards where prisoners are involved.

In addition to satisfying the requirements in section 46.107 of this part, an Institutional Review Board, carrying out responsibilities under this part with respect to research covered by this subpart, shall also meet the following specific requirements:

(a) A majority of the Board (exclusive of prisoner members) shall have no association with the prison(s) involved, apart from their membership on the Board.

(b) At least one member of the Board shall be a prisoner, or a prisoner representative with appropriate background and experience to serve in that capacity, except that where a particular research project is reviewed by more than one Board only one Board need satisfy this requirement.

Section 46.305 Additional duties of the Institutional Review Boards where prisoners are involved.

(a) In addition to all other responsibilities prescribed for Institutional Review Boards under this part, the Board shall review research covered by this subpart and approve such research only if it finds that:

(1) The research under review represents one of the categories of research permissible under section 46.306(a)(2);

(2) Any possible advantages accruing to the prisoner through his or her participation in the research, when compared to the general living conditions, medical care, quality of food, amenities and opportunity for earnings in the prison, are not of such a magnitude that his or her ability to weigh the risks of the research against the value of such advantages in the limited choice environment of the prison is impaired;

(3) The risks involved in the research are commensurate with risks that would be accepted by nonprisoner volunteers;

(4) Procedures for the selection of subjects within the prison are fair to all prisoners and immune from arbitrary intervention by prison authorities or prisoners. Unless the principal investigator provides to the Board justification in writing for following some other procedures, control subjects must be selected randomly from the group of available prisoners who meet the characteristics needed for that particular research project:

(5) The information is presented in language which is understandable to the subject population;

(6) Adequate assurance exists that parole boards will not take into account a prisoner's participation in the research in making decisions regarding parole, and each prisoner is clearly informed in advance that participation in the research will have no effect on his or her parole; and

(7) Where the Board finds there may be a need for follow-up examination or care of participants after the end of their participation, adequate provision has been made for such examination or care, taking into account the varying lengths of individual prisoners' sentences, and for informing participants of this fact.

(b) The Board shall carry out such other duties as may be assigned by the Secretary.

(c) The institution shall certify to the Secretary, in such form and manner as the Secretary may require, that the duties of the Board under this section have been fulfilled.

Section 46.306 Permitted research involving prisoners.

(a) Biomedical or behavioral research conducted or supported by DHHS may involved prisoners as subjects only if:

(1) The institution responsible for the conduct of the research has certified to the Secretary that the Institutional Review Board has approved the research under section 46.305 of this subpart; and

(2) In the judgment of the Secretary the proposed research involves solely the following:

(i) Study the possible causes, effects, and processes of incarceration, and of criminal behavior, provided that the study presents no more than minimal risk and no more than inconvenience to the subjects;

(ii) Study of prisons as institutional structures or of prisoners as incarcerated persons, provided that the study presents no more than minimal risk and no more than inconvenience to the subjects;

(iii) Research on conditions particularly affecting prisoners as a class (for example, vaccine trials and other research on hepatitis which is much more prevalent in prisons than elsewhere; and research on social and psychological problems such as alcoholism, drug addiction and sexual assaults) provided that the study may proceed only after the Secretary has consulted with appropriate experts including experts in penology medicine and ethics, and published notice, in the *Federal Register*, of his intent to approve such research; or

(iv) Research on practices, both innovative and accepted, which have the intent and reasonable probability of improving the health or well-being of the subject. In cases in which those studies require the assignment of prisoners in a manner consistent with protocols approved by the IRB to control groups which may not benefit from the research, the study may proceed only after the Secretary has consulted with appropriate experts, including experts in penology medicine and ethics, and published notice, in the *Federal Register*, of his intent to approve such research.

(b) Except as provided in paragraph (a) of this section, biomedical or behavioral research conducted or supported by DHHS shall not involve prisoners as subjects.

Subpart D--Additional Protections for Children Involved as Subjects in Research.
Source: 48 FR 9818, March 8, 1983.

Section 46.401 To what do these regulations apply?

(a) This subpart applies to all research involving children as subjects, conducted or supported by the Department of Health and Human Services.

(1) This includes research conducted by Department employees, except that each head of an Operating Division of the Department may adopt such nonsubstantive, procedural modifications as may be appropriate from an administrative standpoint.

(2) It also includes research conducted or supported by the Department of Health and Human Services outside the United States, but in appropriate circumstances, the Secretary may, under paragraph (e) of section 46.101 of Subpart A, waive the applicability of some or all of the requirements of these regulations for research of this type.

(b) Exemptions (1), (2), (5) and (6) as listed in Subpart A at section 46.101(b) are applicable to this subpart. Exemption (4), research involving the observation of public behavior, listed at section 46.101(b), is applicable to this subpart where the investigator(s) does not participate in the activities being observed. Exemption (3), research involving survey or interview procedures, listed at section 46.101(b) does not apply to research covered by this subpart.

(c) The exceptions, additions, and provisions for waiver as they appear in paragraphs (c) through (i) of section 46.101 of Subpart A are applicable to this subpart.

Section 46.402 Definitions.

The definitions in section 46.102 of Subpart A shall be applicable to this subpart as well. In addition, as used in this subpart:

(a) "Children" are persons who have not attained the legal age for consent of treatments or procedures involved in the research, under the applicable law of the jurisdiction in which the research will be conducted.

(b) "Assent" means a child's affirmative agreement to participate in research. Mere failure to object should not, absent affirmative agreement, be construed as assent.

(c) "Permission" means the agreement of parent(s) or guardian to the participation of their child or ward in research.

(d) "Parent" means a child's biological or adoptive parent.

(e) "Guardian" means an individual who is authorized under applicable state or local law to consent on behalf of a child to general medical care.

Section 46.403 IRB duties.

In addition to other responsibilities assigned to IRBs under this part, each IRB shall review research covered by this subpart and approve only research which satisfies the conditions of all applicable sections of this subpart.

Section 46.404 Research not involving greater than minimal risk.

HHS will conduct or fund research in which the IRB finds that no greater than minimal risk to children is presented, only if the IRB finds that adequate provisions are made for soliciting the assent of the children and the permission of their parents or guardians, as set forth in section 46.408.

Section 46.405 Research involving greater than minimal risk but presenting the prospect of direct benefit to the individual subjects.

HHS will conduct or fund research in which the IRB finds that more than minimal risk to children is presented by an intervention or procedure that holds out the prospect of direct benefit for the individual subject, or by a monitoring procedure that is likely to contribute to the subject's well-being only if the IRB finds that:

(a) The risk is justified by the anticipated benefit to the subjects;

(b) The relation of the anticipated benefit to the risk is at least as favorable to the subjects as that presented by available alternative approaches; and

(c) Adequate provisions are made for soliciting the assent of the children and permission of their parents or guardians, as set forth in section 46.408.

Section 46.406 Research involving greater than minimal risk and no prospect of direct benefit to individual subjects, but likely to yield generalizable knowledge about the subject's disorder or condition.

HHS will conduct or fund research in which the IRB finds that more than minimal risk to children is presented by an intervention or procedure that does not hold out the prospect of direct benefit for the individual subject, or by a monitoring procedure which is not likely to contribute to the well-being of the subject, only if the IRB finds that:

(a) The risk represents a minor increase over minimal risk;

(b) The intervention or procedure presents experiences to subjects that are reasonably commensurate with those inherent in their actual or expected medical, dental, psychological, social, or educational situations;

(c) The intervention or procedure is likely to yield generalizable knowledge about the subjects' disorder or condition which is of vital importance for the understanding or amelioration of the subjects' disorder or condition; and

(d) Adequate provisions are made for soliciting assent of the children and permission of their parents or guardians, as set forth in section 46.408.

Section 46.407 Research not otherwise approvable which presents an opportunity to understand, prevent, or alleviate a serious problem affecting the health or welfare of children.

HHS will conduct or fund research that the IRB does not believe meets the requirements of sections 46.404, 46.405, or 46.406 only if:

(a) The IRB finds that the research presents a reasonable opportunity to further the understanding, prevention, or alleviation of a serious problem affecting the health or welfare of children; and

(b) The Secretary, after consultation with a panel of experts in pertinent disciplines (for example: science, medicine, education, ethics, law) and following opportunity for public review and comment, has determined either: (1) That the research in fact satisfies the conditions of sections 46.404, 46.405, or 46.406, as applicable, or (2) the following:

(i) The research presents a reasonable opportunity to further the understanding, prevention, or alleviation of a serious problem affecting the health or welfare of children;

(ii) The research will be conducted in accordance with sound ethical principles;

(iii) Adequate provisions are made for soliciting the assent of children and the permission of their parents or guardians, as set forth in section 46.408.

Section 46.408 Requirements for permission by parents or guardians and for assent by children.

(a) In addition to the determinations required under other applicable sections of this subpart, the IRB shall determine that adequate provisions are made for soliciting the assent of the children, when in the judgment of the IRB the children are capable of providing assent. In determining whether children are capable of assenting, the IRB shall take into account the ages, maturity, and psychological state of the children involved. This judgment may be made for all children to be involved in research under a particular protocol, or for each child, as the IRB deems appropriate. If the IRB determines that the capability of some or all of the children is so limited that they cannot reasonably be consulted or that the intervention or procedure involved in the research holds out a prospect of direct benefit that is important to the health or well-being of the children and is available only in the context of the research, the assent of the children is not a necessary condition for proceeding with the research. Even where the IRB determines that the subjects are capable of assenting, the IRB may still waive the assent requirement under circumstances in which consent may be waived in accord with section 46.116 of Subpart A.

(b) In addition to the determinations required under other applicable sections of this subpart, the IRB shall determine, in accordance with and to the extent that consent is required by section 46.116 of Subpart A, that adequate provisions are made for soliciting the permission of each child's parents or guardian. Where parental permission is to be obtained, the IRB may find that the permission of one parent is sufficient for research to be conducted under sections 46.404 or 46.405. Where research is covered by sections 46.406 and 46.407 and permission is to be obtained from parents, both parents must give their permission unless one parent is deceased, unknown, incompetent, or not reasonably available, or when only one parent has legal responsibility for the care and custody of the child.

(c) In addition to the provisions for waiver contained in section 46.116 of Subpart A, if the IRB determines that a research protocol is designed for conditions or for a subject population for which parental or guardian permission is not a reasonable requirement to protect the subjects (for example, neglected or abused children), it may waive the consent requirements in Subpart A of this part and paragraph (b) of this section, provided an appropriate mechanism for protecting the children who will participate as subjects in the research is substituted, and provided further that the waiver is not inconsistent with federal, state or local law. The choice of an appropriate mechanism would depend upon the nature and purpose of the activities described in the protocol, the risk and anticipated benefit to the research subjects, and their age, maturity, status, and condition.

(d) Permission by parents or guardians shall be documented in accordance with and to the extent required by section 46.117 of Subpart A.

(e) When the IRB determines that assent is required, it shall also determine whether and how assent must be documented.

Section 46.409 Wards.

(a) Children who are wards of the state or any other agency, institution, or entity can be included in research approved under sections 46.406 or 46.407 only if such research is:

(1) Related to their status as wards; or

(2) Conducted in schools, camps, hospitals, institutions, or similar settings in which the majority of children involved as subjects are not wards.

(b) If the research is approved under paragraph (a) of this section, the IRB shall require appointment of an advocate for each child who is a ward, in addition to any other individual acting on behalf of the child as guardian or in loco parentis. One individual may serve as advocate for more than one child. The advocate shall be an individual who has the background and experience to act in, and agrees to act in, the best interests of the child for the duration of the child's participation in the research and who is not associated in any way (except in the role as advocate or member of the IRB) with the research, the investigator(s), or the guardian organization.

Notices

Human Subjects: Minimum Criteria Identifying the Viable Fetus

On March 13, 1975, regulations were published in the *Federal Register* (40 FR 11854) relating to the protection of human subjects in research, development, and related activities supported by Department of Health, Education, and Welfare grants and contracts. These regulations are codified at 45 CFR Part 46.

Elsewhere in this issue of the *Federal Register*, the Secretary is amending 45 CFR Part 46 by, among other things, adding a new Subpart B to provide additional protections pertaining to research, development, and related activities involving fetuses, pregnant women, and in vitro fertilization.

Section 46.203(d) of Subpart B provides inter alia as follows:

> The Secretary may from time to time, taking into account medical advances, publish in the *Federal Register* guidelines to assist in determining whether a fetus is viable for purposes of this subpart.

This notice is published in accordance with section 46.203(d). For purposes of Subpart B, the guidelines indicating that a fetus other than a dead fetus within the meaning of section 46.203(f) is viable include the following:

> an estimated gestational age of 20 weeks or more and a body weight of 500 grams or more.

Source: 40 FR 33528, Aug. 8, 1975.

Research Activities Which May Be Reviewed Through Expedited Review Procedures

Research activities involving no more than minimal risk *and* in which the only involvement of human subjects will be in one or more of the following categories (carried out through standard methods) may be reviewed by the Institutional Review Board through the expedited review procedure authorized in 46.110 of 45 CFR Part 46.

1. Collection of: hair and nail clippings, in a nondisfiguring manner; deciduous teeth; and permanent teeth if patient care indicates a need for extraction.
2. Collection of excreta and external secretions including sweat, uncannulated saliva, placenta removed at delivery, and amniotic fluid at the time of rupture of the membrane prior to or during labor.
3. Recording of data from subjects 18 years of age or older using noninvasive procedures routinely employed in clinical practice. This includes the use of physical sensors that are applied either to the surface of the body or at a distance and do not involve input of matter or significant amounts of energy into the subject or an invasion of the subject's privacy. It also includes such procedures as weighing, testing sensory acuity, electrocardiography, electroencephalography, thermography, detection of naturally occurring radioactivity, diagnostic echography, and electroretinography. It does not include exposure to electromagnetic radiation outside the visible range (for example, x-rays, microwaves).
4. Collection of blood samples by venipuncture, in amounts not exceeding 450 milliliters in an eight-week period and no more often than two times per week, from subjects 18 years of age or older and who are in good health and not pregnant.
5. Collection of both supra- and subgingival dental plaque and calculus, provided the procedure is not more invasive than routine prophylactic scaling of the teeth and the process is accomplished in accordance with accepted prophylactic techniques.
6. Voice recordings made for research purposes such as investigations of speech defects.
7. Moderate exercise by healthy volunteers.
8. The study of existing data, documents, records, pathological specimens, or diagnostic specimens.
9. Research on individual or group behavior or characteristics of individuals, such as studies of perception, cognition, game theory, or test development, where the investigator does not manipulate subjects' behavior and the research will not involve stress to subjects.
10. Research on drugs or devices for which an investigational new drug exemption or an investigational device exemption is not required.

Source: 46 FR 8392, Jan. 26, 1981.

Appendix B

A Protocol for Determining Consent Form Readability

The Concept of Readability

Readability testing has been used by educators, in one form or another, for over 40 years. Basically, it is a procedure that will predict the reading grade level required to understand any given document. In most formulas this prediction is accomplished by measuring two variables: the length of the sentences and the complexity of the words. Validation is normally achieved by correlating predicted scores against a series of reading passages that have been calibrated precisely for grade level through extensive field tests.

Readability formulas, however, are not completely free of drawbacks. First, they are not perfect indicators, but are essentially estimates. The error of prediction can range from as little as one-half grade levels to nearly two grade levels. Second, readability tests generally measure only structural difficulty. That is, they will nicely measure such things as sentence structure, vocabulary level, and idea density, but they will not take account of other factors that may influence comprehension, such as the way the material is organized, the circumstances under which it is presented, or a variety of characteristics of the readers.

Currently over 50 different formulas can be used to estimate readability,[1] including formulas for activities ranging from listening to speakers to reading programmed materials, military manuals, and shorthand passages. In addition, there are readability formulas for foreign languages such as French, Dutch, Spanish, Hebrew, German, Hindi, Russian, and Chinese--with additional procedures for Korean, Japanese, Vietnamese, and Thai.

A Suggested Readability Protocol

Here are three procedures that have been found useful in determining the readability levels of consent forms and related explanatory materials. Each procedure has various strengths and weaknesses. However, when used in combination as an evaluative protocol, they provide an excellent system for assessing consent readability.

I recommend that the process begin by using the Flesch Formula[2,3] as an initial indicator of general readability. This formula will place the document in one of five categories of literary difficulty: Academic or Scientific, Quality, Standard, Slick Fiction, or Pulp Fiction. In most situations, if a document scores in either the Academic and Scientific or Quality categories, it will have to be rewritten.

The rewriting process should begin by determining the exact grade level of the material. For this purpose, the Fry Scale[4] should be used. Rewrite the document until the desired grade level, according to the Fry Scale, is achieved. For most purposes, this should be the top of the ninth grade level: *no higher than* 4.5 sentences per 100 words and *less than* 148 syllables per 100 words.

If the forms are extensive in length (i.e., more than 30 sentences) or you are using supplementary booklets or materials, I suggest you use the SMOG Grading System.[5] This system will provide a very fast, easy, and accurate way of determining the readability of documents ranging from a few typed pages to entire books.

One final note: While this section deals primarily with the readability of documents, you must remember that an enormous amount of information is transmitted through your spoken explanation. Not only must your forms and materials be readable, but your presentation must be "listenable." In 1966, Fang[6] did a study of televised newscasts to determine the level at which an oral presentation must be made to be considered desirable for mass listenability. Based on his work, you may want to keep in mind that maximum listenability is obtained when the number of syllables above one per word in a sentence is kept below 12.

The Readability Formulas

The Flesch Readability Formula

Step 1: Collect three 100-word samples from the consent form, either from the beginning, middle, and end of the document or from specific important segments (e.g., the purpose, procedure, and risk/discomfort sections). If the form is less than 300 words, you may collect fewer samples, but be sure you are collecting enough to make a fair test. Each sample should start at the beginning of a paragraph, if possible. Count contractions and hyphenated words as one word. Count as words all numbers or letters separated by a space.

Step 2: Count the total syllables in each of your 100-word samples. When counting syllables in figures, count them the way they are read aloud, i.e., 1986 would be "nine-teen eigh-ty six." If there are numerous or lengthy figures in

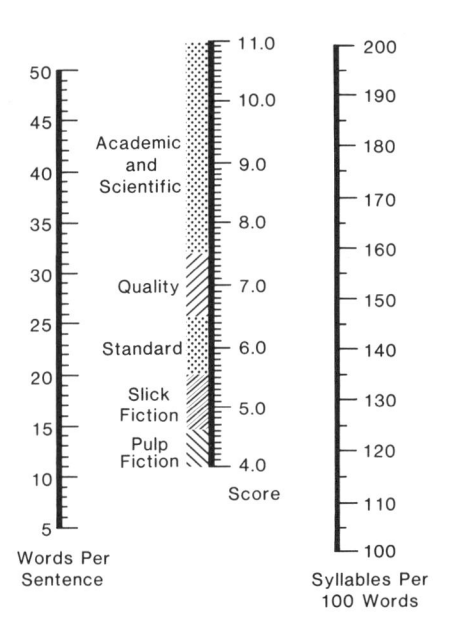

Figure 1 Flesch-Powers Nomogram

Source: Powers, R. D., and J. E. Ross. "New Diagrams for Calculating Readability Scores Rapidly." *Journalism Quarterly* 36 (1959):177-182. Reprinted by permission.

your passage, your estimate will be more accurate if you don't include them. However, be sure to add a corresponding number of words to the end of your sample. Any good dictionary, of course, will provide syllabication rules if you are in doubt. One simple way to speed the process of syllable counting is to select a key on an electric typewriter--let's say the letter "l"--and read the passage to yourself, tapping out the number of syllables in each word on the typewriter key. When you have completed the passage, simply block out by "fives" the number of l's you have typed, count them up, and this will be your total syllable count. Next, average the syllable counts from each of your three passages. This figure will be the "average syllables per 100 words" for that document.

Step 3: Next figure the average sentence length of your passage. In each of your samples find the sentence that ends nearest the 100-word mark. (This sentence could end, for example, on the 94th word, or it could end on the 190th word.) Count the total number of sentences in your sample (up to that point) and divide this figure into the total number of words in your sample (up to that point). Average this result from each of your three samples as you did in step two. This number is the "average words per sentence" for that document.

Step 4: The final step is to turn to Figure 1. Plot the average words per sentence (Step 3) on the left scale and the average syllables per 100 words

(Step 2) on the right scale. Next, draw a line connecting these two plotted points. The readability of your consent form can be read at the point this line crosses the middle figure.

As you can see, this middle figure is divided into five categories corresponding to various degrees of difficulty. The approximate literary equivalents of these categories can be seen in Table 1:

Table 1

LITERARY EQUIVALENTS OF FLESCH/POWERS
READABILITY CATEGORIES

Flesch Category	Literary Equivalent
Academic and Scientific	*Science, Yale Review, Harvard Educational Review*
Quality	*Harper's, Atlantic Monthly*
Standard	*Reader's Digest, Time, Newsweek*
Slick Fiction	*Colliers, Ladies' Home Journal, Good Housekeeping*
Pulp Fiction	*True Confessions*

The Fry Readability Scale

Step 1: Collect three 100-word samples from the consent form, either from the beginning, middle, and end of the document or from specific important segments (e.g., the purpose, procedure, and risk/discomfort sections). If the form is less than 300 words, you may collect fewer samples, but be sure you are collecting enough to make a fair test. Skip all proper nouns.

Step 2: Count the total number of sentences in each 100-word passage. If the sample ends in the middle of a sentence, estimate to the nearest tenth of a sentence. Average these numbers from your three samples. This is the "average number of sentences per 100 words" for this document.

Step 3: Count the total number of syllables in each 100-word sample as you did in Step 2 of the Flesch Formula. Again, it is recommended that the typewriter keying technique be used. Average these numbers. This is the "average number of syllables per 100 words" for this document.

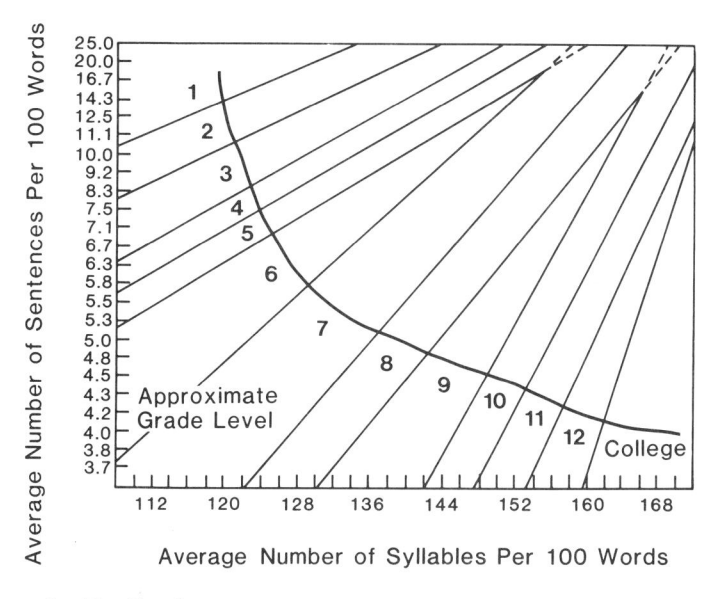

Figure 2 Fry Graph

Source: E. A. Fry. "A Readability Formula that Saves Time." *Journal of Reading* 11 (1968):513-516.

Step 4: To obtain the grade level equivalency of your document, simply plot the average number of sentences per 100 words (Step 2) on the axis and the average number of syllables per 100 words (Step 3) on the abscissa of the graph provided in Figure 2. The approximate grade-level equivalency can be read off the curved line. The grade level which is appropriate for your consent form is, of course, dependent upon the population for which it is intended. You may want to keep in mind, however, that other general consumption documents, such as newspapers, are written at about a seventh or eighth grade level.

SMOG Grading

Step 1: Count 10 consecutive sentences near the beginning of the text, 10 in the middle, and 10 near the end. Count as a sentence any string of words ending with a period, a question mark, or exclamation point.

Step 2: In the 30 selected sentences, count every word of three or more syllables. Any string of letters or numerals beginning and ending with a space or punctuation mark should be counted if you can distinguish at least three syllables when you read it aloud in context. If a polysyllabic word is repeated, count each repetition.

Step 3: Calculate the square root of the total number of polysyllabic words counted. (If a calculator is not handy and the reader does not wish to do the calculation in long hand, an estimation process is possible. This is done by taking the square root of the nearest perfect square. For example, if the count is 95, the nearest perfect square is 100, which yields a perfect square of 10. If the count lies roughly between two perfect squares, choose the lower number. For instance, if the count is 110, take the square root of 100 rather than 121).

Step 4: Add 3 to the square root you calculated in Step 3. This gives you the SMOG grade, which is the reading grade level that a person must have reached if he is to fully understand the document tested.

If the consent form or document contains less than 30 sentences, and you still wish to use the SMOG system, follow these procedures:

1. Count the number of polysyllabic words in the entire text.
2. Count the total number of sentences in the entire text.
3. Divide the total number of polysyllabic words by the total number of sentences.
4. Multiply this average by the number of sentences you are short of 30.
5. Add that figure to the total number of polysyllabic words.
6. Find the square root of that figure and add the constant 3.

You may want to keep in mind, however, that the accuracy of the SMOG grade goes down the further your total number of sentences is from 30. Thus, if you are seriously short of 30 sentences, you may wish to use the Fry Scale to obtain the grade-level equivalency of your consent form.

References

1. Klare, G. R. "Assessing Readability." *Reading Research Quarterly* 10 (1974):62-102.

2. Flesch, R. "A New Readability Yardstick." *Journal of Applied Psychology* 32 (1948):221-233.

3. Powers, R. D., and J. E. Ross. "New Diagrams for Calculating Readability Scores Rapidly." *Journalism Quarterly* 36 (1959):177-182.

4. Fry, E. A. "A Readability Formula That Saves Time." *Journal of Reading* 11 (1968):513-516.

5. McLaughlin, G. H. "SMOG Grading--A New Readability Formula." *Journal of Reading* 12 (1969): 639-646.

6. "The Easy Listening Formula." *Journal of Broadcasting* 11 (1966):63-68.

Appendix C

Sample Consent Form Rewrite

Rewrite of Consent Form Found on Page 95

*Reading Equivalency = 7th to 8th Grade**

The Institute for Counseling Services is doing a study of ways to control anxiety. We want to see if a new method called biofeedback will work. We know it works on high school students. We want to see if it will work on test anxiety in college freshmen. This will involve you in six one-hour sessions each about one week apart. We hope to use these data to improve the counseling program at West Overshoe Tech.

At these sessions an experienced staff member will show you what to do. You will be attached to a device that will make clicking sounds. These sounds will tell you how tense or relaxed your muscles are. Your job will be to sit back, relax, and try to make the clicking sounds decrease in number. There are no known risks or discomforts connected with doing this. We think this method may be of great help in treating test anxiety. If you decide not to be a part of the study, however, you will still have access to all the regular counseling services.

All information will be kept secret. While we might write about the study, your name will never be used. You can quit anytime you want without problems. If you have any questions after today, please feel free to call Dr. Smyth at 555-3801.

I, _____, have read this statement and have had all my questions answered.

Date: _____

Signature: _____

Witness: _____

---

* *Flesch*: Slick Fiction (e.g., *Good Housekeeping*, *Ladies' Home Journal*, etc.). *Fry*: Low 7th Grade. *SMOG*: 8.16 (Score may be problematic, however, due to inadequate number of sentences.)

Appendix D

A Consent Checklist

As in the main body of this text, the numbers in brackets refer to items that are mandated by 45 CFR 46.

I. Preliminaries

Yes   No

_____   _____   1. Does the project, according to the definitions in 45 CFR 46, propose to conduct "research" on "human subjects"? [46.102(e) and (f)] (If no, stop here. No consent is needed.)

_____   _____   2. Is the consent form likely to be understandable to the intended subject population as tested by a readability formula? [46.116]

_____   _____   3. If a "short form" is being used, has provision been made for a witness to attend each consent session? [46.117(b)(2)]

II. Consent Execution

Yes   No

_____   _____   1. Were two copies of the consent form passed out to the subjects? [46.117]

_____   _____   2. Was the consent form read out loud as the subjects silently read along?

_____ _____ 3. Was a brief verbal summary given to the subjects after the reading?

_____ _____ 4. Did the experimenter ask for questions?

_____ _____ 5. Was a reasonable opportunity given for the subjects to consider whether to participate? [46.116]

_____ _____ 6. Was there any evidence that the subjects were lied to or in any way forced, coerced, or deceived into signing the consent form? [46.116]

_____ _____ 7. Were the subjects asked to sign and date both copies of the consent form? [46.117]

_____ _____ 8. Were the subjects instructed to keep one copy of the consent form for their own records? [46.117]

_____ _____ 9. Were those who did not sign dismissed in a friendly and courteous manner?

III. The Consent Form

Yes   No

_____ _____ 1. Does the consent form state who is doing the experiment?

_____ _____ 2. Does the consent form state the nature, purpose, and duration of the experiment, including the fact that it is experimental? [46.116(a)(1)]

_____ _____ 3. Does the consent form state the uses to be made of the data?

_____ _____ 4. Does the consent form state the procedures to be employed in the experiment? [46.116(a)(1)]

_____ _____ 5. Does the consent form state the hazards, inconveniences, and risks the subject will undergo, so far as they are known? [46.116(a)(2)]

_____ _____ 6. If appropriate, does the consent form state the availability of compensation and treatment if the subject is injured? [46.116(a)(6)]

_____ _____ 7. Does the consent form state the benefits that might be expected? [46.116(a)(3)]

_____ _____ 8. Does the consent form, if the experiment is therapeutically related, disclose the alternate procedures the subject may choose? [46.116(a)(4)]

_____ _____ 9. Does the consent form state the conditions of participation, if any? [46.116(b)(4)]

_____ _____ 10. Does the consent form contain a statement of the extent to which the confidentiality of the data will be maintained? [46.116(a)(5)]

_____ _____ 11. If appropriate, does the consent form describe the procedures to be employed in maintaining confidentiality?

_____ _____ 12. Does the consent form mention that the subject is at liberty to withdraw his or her prior consent to the experiment or discontinue participation in the experiment at any time without prejudice? [46.116(a)(8)]

_____ _____ 13. Does the consent form contain instructions as to who and how to contact someone if questions or problems should arise later on? [46.116(a)(7)]

_____ _____ 14. Does the consent document contain any exculpatory language? [46.116]

_____ _____ 15. Is there a place for the date of signing and for the signature of the subject and witness? [46.117(b)(1)-(2)]

IV. Additional Inclusions

Yes   No

_____ _____ 1. If appropriate, does the consent form state that the procedure may involve unforeseeable risks? [46.116(b)(1)]

_____ _____ 2. If appropriate, does the consent form state that any significant new findings affecting risk will be reported to the subject? [46.116(b)(5)]

Yes	No	
_____	_____	3. If appropriate, does the consent form state the circumstances under which the experimenter may terminate the subject's participation? [46.116(b)(2)]
_____	_____	4. If appropriate, does the consent form state any possible additional costs the subject may have to bear? [46.116(b)(3)]
_____	_____	5. If appropriate, does the consent form state the consequences of the subject's withdrawal from the study? [46.116(b)(4)]
_____	_____	6. If appropriate, does the consent form state the approximate number of subjects in the study? [46.116(b)(6)]

V. Altering or Waiving the Consent Process

Yes	No	
		(Note: The answers to questions 1 to 3 must all be "no" and the answer to 4 must be "yes" for alteration or waiver approval to be given.)
_____	_____	1. Does the research involve greater than minimal risk? [46.116(d)(1)]
_____	_____	2. Will the alteration or waiver adversely affect the rights or welfare of the subjects? [46.116(d)(2)]
_____	_____	3. Practically speaking, could the research be carried out without the waiver or alteration? [46.116(d)(3)]
_____	_____	4. If possible, will the subjects be provided with additional pertinent information after participation? [46.116(d)(4)]

VI. Altering or Waiving Consent Documentation

Yes	No	
		(Note: The answers to questions 1 and 2 must be "yes"; *or*, the answers to questions 3 and 4 must be "no" for an alteration or waiver approval to be given.)

_____ _____ 1. Is the consent form the only record linking the subject to the research and could it potentially be harmful to the subject if the confidentiality of the research were breached? [46.117(c)(1)]

_____ _____ 2. Will each subject be asked if he or she wants documentation linking him or her to the research? [46.117(c)(1)]

_____ _____ 3. Does the research involve more than minimal risk? [46.117(c)(2)]

_____ _____ 4. Does the research involve any procedures for which written consent is normally required outside of the research context? [46.117(c)(2)]